Arthritis

CHU
LIVII

Churchill Livingstone
An imprint of Elsevier Limited.

 is a registered trademark of Elsevier Limited.

© 2004 Elsevier Limited.

The right of Gabriel Panayi and D John Dickson to be identified as the authors
of this Work has been asserted by them in accordance with the Copyright,
Designs and Patents Act 1988.

ISBN 0443 074674

Cataloguing in Publication Data
Catalogue records for this book are available from the US Library of Congress
and the British Library.

Note
Medical knowledge is constantly changing. As new information becomes
available, changes in treatment, procedures, equipment and the use of drugs
become necessary. The authors and the publishers have taken care to ensure that
the information given in this text is accurate and up to date. However, readers
are strongly advised to confirm that the information, especially with regard to
drug usage, complies with the latest legislation and standards of practice.

Printed in China

Contents

Preface

Diseases of the musculoskeletal system are responsible for a huge amount of pain and suffering. We hope that *In Clinical Practice: Arthritis* will serve an important role in educating and guiding current and future primary care health professionals in treating musculoskeletal diseases. The breadth of patients seen in primary care is phenomenal and musculoskeletal medicine accounts for around 25% of the primary care workload. Primary care refers about 17% of these patients to secondary care.

The aim of this book is to supply guidance and knowledge to doctors and other health professionals when managing these patients so that the most effective treatment and advice can be given. For those patients who are managed within primary care, it is about the practical and the possible rather than the impossible ideal. For patients who may need secondary care, the aim is to help doctors decide which patients to refer to a rheumatologist, the facilities offered in secondary care, the main disease entities within the remit of the consultant rheumatologist and general practice monitoring of a patient under secondary care.

The training of doctors is mainly focused around university hospitals and their consultants, with comparatively little time spent in the primary care environment despite the fact that, today, more and more emphasis is placed on managing patients in primary care. It is hoped that this book will be a useful adjunct for primary care physicians, tutors and their colleagues as well as medical students. It should prove invaluable for Primary Care Trusts that are developing musculoskeletal clinics with special interest and for extended scope physiotherapists and nurse practitioners.

Gabriel Panayi
D John Dickson

Biographies

Professor Gabriel S Panayi ScD, MD, FRCP is Arthritis Research Campaign Professor of Rheumatology in the Department of Rheumatology, Guy's, King's and St Thomas' School of Medicine, King's College London and honorary consultant in rheumatology at Guy's and St Thomas' Hospital, London. His clinical interests are in the inflammatory rheumatic diseases, especially rheumatoid arthritis. His major research interests are the pathogenesis and immunotherapy of rheumatoid arthritis. He has been President of the British Society of Rheumatology and President of the Clinical Immunology and Allergy Section of the Royal Society of Medicine, London. He has received numerous honours and prizes including Heberden Orator of the British Society of Rheumatology. He founded the European Workshop for Rheumatology Research in 1981 and has written or edited several books on rheumatology as well as contributing chapters in books and review articles. His published scientific work consists of more than 300 refereed papers.

D John Dickson MB ChB, FRCP (Glas), FRCP (Lond), MRCGP is a general practitioner in Yorkshire and co-founder and Business Manager of the Primary Care Rheumatology (PCR) Society, which provides education and resources to help general practitioners manage patients with arthritis. He helped lead the Society's National Institute for Clinical Excellence (NICE) submissions on Cox-2 and tumour necrosis factor (TNF) alpha drugs. He now commits his time mainly to primary care rheumatology, running musculoskeletal clinics for Langbaurgh PCT. He is a member of the Education committee for the Arthritis Research Campaign and editor of their publication "In Practice", which has now been superseded by a new publication "Hands On", distributed to all general practitioners in the UK. Together with Dr Gillian Hosie (past President of the PCR), he has written a question and answer book for doctors, health professionals and patients entitled *Your Questions Answered – Osteoarthritis*.

The big picture

Musculoskeletal disorders are a very important component of a general practitioner's (GP's) workload; 19.5% of a GP's workload is due to musculoskeletal conditions.

General points about arthritis

- 103 million European citizens have arthritis/rheumatism. They comprise the largest part of the population living with a long-term medical condition.
- Arthritis affects an estimated 42.7 million Americans (nearly 1 in 6 people).
- Arthritis limits over 7 million Americans from participating in their main daily activities such as going to work or maintaining their independence.
- More than 7 million adults in the UK (15% of the population) have long-term health problems due to arthritis and related conditions.
- Almost 9 million people in the UK (19% of the population) visited their GP in the past year with arthritis and related conditions.
- Two-thirds of people with arthritis (66%) are satisfied with the level of care and treatment they receive from their GP.
- Arthritis and related conditions are the second most common cause of days off work in both men and women.
- Almost nine-tenths of people with arthritis or joint pain (87%) are not under the care of a rheumatologist or orthopaedic surgeon.

Osteoarthritis

- More than 2 million people visited their GP in the past year because of osteoarthritis (OA). The number of people with OA has risen over the past 10 years as the population ages, and more people are now seeking their GP's help.
- At least 4.4 million people in the UK have X-ray evidence of moderate to severe OA in their hands; 550,000 have moderate to severe OA in their knees; and 210,000 have moderate to severe OA of the hips.
- Obesity is a major risk factor for OA of the knee. The UK currently has the eighth highest obesity rate in the world, and numbers are rising.
- More than 44,000 hip replacements and more than 35,000 knee replacements were performed in the UK in 2000.
- 50% of people with arthritis say the worst aspect is pain. This rises to 55% of people with OA.

Rheumatoid arthritis

- Around 387,000 people in the UK have rheumatoid arthritis (RA), roughly 0.8% of the adult population.

"19.5% of a GP's workload is due to musculoskeletal conditions"

"Arthritis and related conditions are the second most common cause of days off work in both men and women"

"Obesity is a major risk factor for osteoarthritis of the knee. The UK currently has the eighth highest obesity rate in the world, and numbers are rising"

"Around 387,000 people in the UK have rheumatoid arthritis, roughly 0.8% of the adult population"

66 Around 2.6 million people in the UK visited their GP with back pain in the past year 99

- There are around 12,000 new cases a year.
- The number of people with RA fell during the 1970s and 1980s but incidence rates have been steady for the past 10 years.

Back pain
- Around 2.6 million people in the UK visited their GP with back pain in the past year.

Rarer conditions
- Around 12,000 children have juvenile idiopathic arthritis in the UK.
- Each year, 200,000 people visit their GP with ankylosing spondylitis.
- Each year, around 250,000 people with gout visit their GP.
- Around 10,000 people in the UK have systemic lupus erythematosus (SLE).

66 NHS expenditure on arthritis increased by only 5% between 1990 and 1999, compared with an increase of 19% in the total NHS budget 99

The cost to the nation of arthritis and related conditions
- The cost of arthritis in the USA is $65 billion per year, equivalent to a constant, moderate national recession.
- It involves 39 million doctor visits per year.
- 206 million working days were lost in the UK in 1999–2000.
- £2.4 billion was paid in incapacity benefit in 2001.
- £98 million was paid to people claiming severe disablement allowance in 2001.
- Cost of community and social services was £389 million and £1.3 billion, respectively, in 2001.
- National Health Service (NHS) expenditure on arthritis increased by only 5% between 1990 and 1999, compared with an increase of 19% in the total NHS budget.
- Cost of GP consultations was £307 million in 2000.
- Cost of drugs prescribed was £341 million in 2000.
- Costs of rheumatology in hospitals was £259 million in 2000.
- Cost of hip and knee replacements was £405 million in 2000.
- These costs total £5.5 billion in 1 year.

66 These costs total £5.5 billion in one year 99

These figures speak for themselves, attesting to the huge cost (social, economic and personal) imposed by musculoskeletal conditions.

Musculoskeletal conditions clearly need a better framework for diagnosis and management, more resources and, for the more serious conditions at least (RA, inflammatory arthritides and connective tissue diseases [CTDs]), to be made priorities within the NHS.

The vast majority of musculoskeletal disorders are self-limiting. A minority of patients who have more serious disease or chronic disease require specialist referral and management. It is particularly important with chronic disease that the GP and rheumatologist establish a proper cooperative working relationship. This book outlines the important conditions that are met within primary care and discusses the various ways in which secondary care can impact the work in general practice.

Reasons for referral to rheumatology clinics

Most patients with musculoskeletal disorders pose very simple diagnostic and management problems and do not require hospital referral. Reasons for referral to rheumatology clinics include:

- diagnostic uncertainty,
- management uncertainty,
- uncontrolled symptoms,
- increasing disability or deformity,
- disease complications,
- patient or family anxiety, and
- patient demand for a specialist opinion.

The presence of "red flags" in the patient is a useful guide in deciding whether referral is necessary. Red flags include:

- inflamed joint with fever or constitutional disturbance,
- extreme pain or difficulty moving a joint or joints,
- undiagnosed acute inflammatory arthritis,
- severe pain at rest or at night,
- pain that is progressively worse over a period of days or weeks, and
- serious underlying pathology such as a bone tumour or metastasis.

The skills of a rheumatologist

A rheumatologist not only has skills and knowledge in the more serious musculoskeletal diseases, particularly of the connective tissues and inflammatory diseases of the joints, but also a number of special investigative and treatment services that supplement the care provided by the GP.

- Diagnosis
  - skills in clinical examination,
  - synovial fluid,
  - interpretation of immunological tests,
  - access to special imaging technologies,
  - tissue biopsy,
  - experience of rare rheumatic disorders, and
  - the impact of systemic and other diseases on the musculoskeletal system.
- Treatment
  - counselling, educational and self-help programmes,
  - a therapeutic team of physiotherapists, occupational therapists and nurses,

66 Most patients with musculoskeletal disorders pose very simple diagnostic and management problems and do not require hospital referral 99

- admission for hospital in-patient treatment,
- aspiration and injection of joint and soft tissues,
- knowledge of disease-modifying and immunosuppressive drugs and newer treatment modalities including biologics, and
- special therapeutic interventions such as joint lavage, steroid or immunosuppressive pulse therapy, and experimental agents.

The term musculoskeletal conditions includes all conditions that affect the bones, joints and ligaments such as arthritis of all kinds, CTDs, back pain, osteoporosis, soft-tissue rheumatism and regional and widespread pain. The human cost of arthritis and related conditions is huge.

Which conditions will be seen by GPs?

66 The history and clinical examination of a patient presenting with musculoskeletal problems are the bedrock on which further investigation, management and outcome depend 99

Pain in the neck, knee, hip and shoulder and problems with the elbow, wrist, thumb, hand, ankle and foot are important conditions commonly seen by GPs. Both primary and secondary care may be involved in providing care to patients with OA, chronic pain, fibromyalgia, hypermobility and musculoskeletal problems in children, teenagers and the active elderly. Conditions that are generally managed in secondary care include rheumatoid arthritis, crystal arthritis, the seronegative spondyloarthropathies (ankylosing spondylitis and psoriatic arthritis), CTDs (including primary Sjögren's syndrome [SjS]), polymyalgia rheumatica and giant cell arteritis.

Arthritis

History and examination

The history and clinical examination of a patient presenting with musculoskeletal problems are the bedrock on which further investigation, management and outcome depend. The history depends on the patient as a witness but must also be guided by the intelligent use of the doctor's knowledge of musculoskeletal conditions. The clinical examination is guided by the differential diagnosis established during the history-taking process. It vitally contributes to the listing and ranking of the differential diagnoses on which investigations are based and, hopefully, the final diagnosis is made.

Since musculoskeletal conditions can present in innumerable ways and since other conditions, for example metastatic malignancies, can present with musculoskeletal symptoms, history taking can be a long and complex process. However, certain principles can be used in order to focus and simplify history taking.

66 Acute arthritis presenting over a matter of hours or a few days is likely to suggest infective arthritis, or crystal arthritides such as gout or pseudogout 99

Tempo of onset

Acute arthritis presenting over a matter of hours or a few days is likely to suggest infective arthritis or crystal arthritides such as gout or

Tempo of onset of arthritis
Acute • infective arthritis • crystal arthritis **Chronic/insidious** • rheumatoid arthritis • other arthritides • osteoarthritis

Fig. 1 Tempo of onset of arthritis

Number of joints involved
Single (mono) or a few (oligoarticular arthritis) • infective arthritis • osteoarthritis knee(s), hips • ankylosing spondylitis • psoriatic arthritis • reactive arthritis • inflammatory bowel disease **Many joints (polyarticular)** • rheumatoid arthritis • primary generalized osteoarthritis

Fig. 2 Number of joints involved

❝ Rheumatoid arthritis usually presents as a polyarthritis, although the number of joints involved increases with time. The maximum number of joints involved is usually reached early in the course of the disease ❞

pseudogout. A more chronic onset of arthritis can be suggestive of a large number of other conditions including inflammatory diseases such as RA, various forms of oligoarthritis and even OA (Fig. 1).

Number of joints involved

Fig. 2 shows the differential diagnosis according to the number of joints involved. Arthritis presenting acutely in a single joint would suggest crystal arthritis or infection or, occasionally, the presentation of a rheumatoid factor (RF) negative (seronegative) arthritis in association with ankylosing spondylitis, psoriatic arthritis or the peripheral arthritis of inflammatory bowel disease. RA in adults rarely presents in this manner.

Polyarthritic presentation

RA usually presents as a polyarthritis, although the number of joints involved increases with time. The maximum number of joints involved is usually reached early in the course of the disease. Polyarticular disease is also characteristic of primary generalized OA. The distinction between these two conditions is usually clear both in terms of the history, the physical findings and the investigations (detailed below).

Fig. 3 Duration of arthritis

Duration of arthritis
Short duration – days • crystal arthritis • gout • pseudogout **Chronic** • rheumatoid arthritis • primary generalized arthritis • arthritis of seronegative type • ankylosing spondylitis • psoriatic arthritis • reactive arthritis • inflammatory bowel disease

Certain characteristic articular presentations need to be borne in mind: distal interphalangeal joint involvement in patients with psoriatic arthritis and distal interphalangeal joint involvement (Heberden's nodes) in patients with OA. The distinction between the soft tissue swelling in the former and the hard bony swelling in the latter is easy to make on clinical examination.

66 The diurnal pattern of arthritic symptoms is critical in making a correct diagnosis 99

Duration of arthritis
Attacks of arthritis that last a few days and are accompanied by clinical evidence of acute inflammation are usually due to crystal arthritides such as gout and pseudogout. Acute arthritides that may last for longer include infective arthritis and mono- or oligoarthritis of the seronegative arthritides such as ankylosing spondylitis and related conditions. Viral arthritides may fall into this category but the diagnosis is rarely made directly.

Chronic arthritides
The chronic arthritides resolve themselves into RA (symmetrical polyarthritis) or primary generalized OA that involves many of the small joints of the hands, the metatarsophalangeal (MTP) joints of the big toes in the feet and large joint arthritis, particularly in the knees (Fig. 3). Outside these diseases, chronic arthritides occur rarely and are seen as variant forms of SLE and in primary SjS.

Diurnal pattern of arthritic symptoms
The diurnal pattern of arthritic symptoms is critical in making a correct diagnosis.

Inflammatory arthritis characterized by worse symptoms
in the mornings

In the inflammatory arthritides, there is a very distinct diurnal pattern.
Patients have severe symptoms of early morning stiffness and pain and
loss of function on awakening that typically lasts for more than 45
minutes. Many have disturbed sleep because of the increased inflammation at night, typically waking between 3.00am and 4.00am. This is

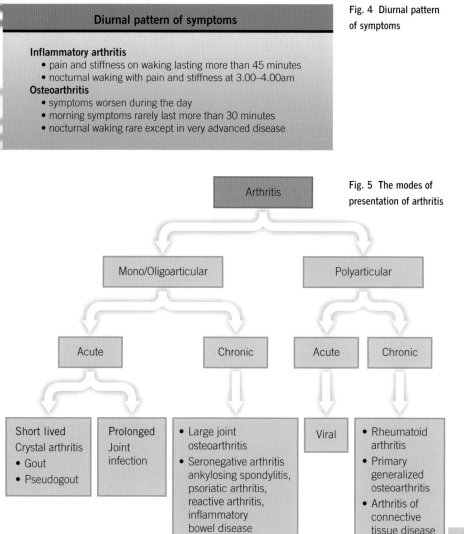

Diurnal pattern of symptoms

Inflammatory arthritis
- pain and stiffness on waking lasting more than 45 minutes
- nocturnal waking with pain and stiffness at 3.00–4.00am

Osteoarthritis
- symptoms worsen during the day
- morning symptoms rarely last more than 30 minutes
- nocturnal waking rare except in very advanced disease

Fig. 4 Diurnal pattern of symptoms

Fig. 5 The modes of presentation of arthritis

13

an important point to remember, as some of these patients may not have early morning stiffness on awakening.

Non-inflammatory arthritis symptoms worse by the end of the day
By contrast, patients with OA may have pain and stiffness in the involved joints in the mornings but this rarely lasts more than 30 minutes. Morning symptoms lasting in excess of 45 minutes should warn one of the possibility of an inflammatory joint disorder. Symptoms of OA become progressively worse during the day, reaching a maximum intensity by evening. Patients with OA are very rarely woken at night, but complain of an inability to fall asleep because of pain when turning in bed. These crucial differences are shown in Fig. 4.

Arthritis diagnostic flow chart
Fig. 5 summarises the modes of presentation of arthritis. The primary divisions are between mono- or oligoarticular versus polyarticular arthritis, and these two forms can be divided into arthritides of acute onset or insidious and chronic onset. The rarer forms of arthritis need not concern us here. These diagnostic categories cover the overwhelming majority of arthritides that are likely to be seen in primary care.

Fig. 6 Tempo of onset
of spinal symptoms

Tempo of onset of spinal symptoms

Acute
- prolapsed intervertebral disc
- vertebral collapse
- metastatic disease

Chronic
- inflammatory spinal disease (spondylitis)
- non-inflammatory degenerative spinal disease (spondylosis)

Fig. 7 Diurnal pattern
of spinal disease

Diurnal pattern of spinal disease

Spondylitis
- pain and stiffness on waking lasting more than 45 minutes
- nocturnal waking with pain and stiffness at 3.00–4.00am

Spondylosis
- symptoms worsen during the day
- morning symptoms rarely last more than 30 minutes
- nocturnal waking rare

Metastatic disease
- persistent pain
- nocturnal pain

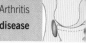

Nevertheless, if arthritis presents with a picture that is not immediately recognisable, referral to a rheumatologist would be indicated.

Spinal disease

Spinal disease is a common manifestation of musculoskeletal disorders. The two most common conditions are cervical and lumbar spondylosis. The inflammatory spinal diseases differ in many important respects from these degenerative conditions. These differences are crucial in establishing the correct diagnosis. The third category of spinal disease that is relevant is that of metastatic spinal disease.

The tempo of the onset of spinal pain is important in establishing the diagnosis (Fig. 6), as is the diurnal pattern (Fig. 7).

Acute spinal disease
Acute spinal pain can be present in the cervical, dorsal or lumbar spines.

Cervical spine
Acute presentation of cervical spine pain is not unusual. It may be accompanied by radicular symptoms and signs down one arm or, occasionally, both arms. The pain may last for some days or even weeks. A patient presenting with symptoms and neurological signs of radicular involvement requires immediate diagnostic workup. Other rarer pathologies may be involved but these will only be uncovered on diagnostic imaging.

Dorsal spine
The most common reason for acute pain in the dorsal spine is osteoporotic vertical collapse or metastatic disease. There may be radicular symptoms radiating to the ribs on one or both sides. Particular attention should be paid to patients who have nocturnal dorsal spinal pain as this may be indicative of metastatic disease but can also happen with osteoporotic collapse or ankylosing spondylitis.

Lumbar spine
Acute pain in the lumbar spine is the common presentation of low back pain. Pain may be localized to the lumbar spine or may radiate to one or other buttock or more extensively down the legs in the distribution of the femoral or sciatic nerves. Pain that worsens on coughing or straining is indicative of a space-occupying lesion, usually a prolapsed intervertebral disc. Metastatic lumbar spinal disease can present acutely, as will lumbar vertebral collapse. In both these situations there may or may not be a radicular distribution of pain. Patients with sphincteric disturbance should be referred immediately to either a neurologist or a rheumatologist.

❝ Spinal disease is a common manifestation of musculoskeletal disorders ❞

❝ Red Flag: Patients with sphincteric disturbance should be referred immediately to either a neurologist or a rheumatologist ❞

Chronic spinal presentation

> *Diseases that present in a chronic and persistent fashion are divided into the inflammatory spinal diseases (spondylitis), and the non-inflammatory spinal diseases, (spondylosis)*

Diseases that present in a chronic and persistent fashion are divided into the inflammatory spinal diseases (spondylitis), and the non-inflammatory spinal disease (spondylosis).

Inflammatory spinal disease

> *Inflammatory spinal diseases characteristically present mainly in young males*

These diseases characteristically present mainly in young males. These patients often have a family history of psoriasis, inflammatory bowel disease or spondylitic disease and they may present with psoriasis or inflammatory bowel disease or even a previous bout of uveitis. They characteristically awake with pain and stiffness in the spine, which may include the cervical, dorsal or lumbar spine. They complain of lack of movement and discomfort. Symptoms may improve during the day but worsen in the evening. They may awaken in the small hours of the night with spinal pain and stiffness and usually get out of bed, walk around for a time to relieve the stiffness, and then go back to bed to sleep until the normal waking time. On occasions, the spondylitis may present with an additional history of radicular symptoms in the neck radiating down an arm, in the dorsal spine radiating along the ribs, or in the lumbar spine radiating along some part or occasionally all of the territory of the femoral or sciatic nerve. The pain is cough impulse negative.

Spondylosis

The symptoms of degenerative spinal disease, whether in the cervical or lumbar spine, worsen during the day. Morning symptoms of pain and stiffness rarely last more than 30 minutes and nocturnal waking is uncommon. Radicular symptoms are unusual unless an acute episode is superimposed on chronic disease.

Metastatic spinal disease

This is characterized by persistent pain associated with nocturnal pain. There may be other evidence of malignant disease such as weight loss and symptoms referable to the tumour itself, although these may be absent.

Connective tissue diseases

The CTDs are important because they may have a bad prognosis. Their prevalence is low so the average GP is unlikely to meet more than the occasional case in a professional lifetime. Nevertheless, it is important to consider them as there are certain aspects that may lead one to suspect that such a disease may be present. The following CTDs will be considered here and later in the book:

- primary SjS,
- SLE,

Some aspects of the symptomatology of connective tissue disorders

• Raynaud's phenomenon
• systemic features
  – anorexia
  – weight loss
  – fever
• skin rashes on sun-exposed parts of the body; other rashes
• loss of hair
• venous or arterial thromboses
• muscle weakness

Fig. 8 Some aspects of the symptomatology of connective tissue disorders

- scleroderma,
- myositis,
- antiphospholipid syndrome.

Some aspects of the symptomatology of connective tissue disorders are summarised in Fig. 8. Raynaud's phenomenon is common to many of these conditions. It is important to obtain the description of a triphasic colour response in the fingers and/or the toes consisting of normal skin followed by whiteness of the skin and then a hyperaemic phase when the skin goes blue or red followed by a return to normal colour. Many patients have systemic features such as anorexia, weight loss or fever. A variety of rashes may be present but particularly characteristic are ultraviolet-sensitive skin rashes on some exposed parts of the body. Many patients may lose hair. There may be venous or arterial thromboses with a complex symptomatology including deep vein thrombosis in the leg presenting with pain and swelling of the calf. This may be followed by shortness of breath and chest pain caused by pulmonary embolism. Arterial thromboses may present in a number of ways including stroke. Proximal muscle weakness with tenderness may be the presenting symptom of myositis. Finally, recurrent abortions may be a feature of women with SLE, particularly if they are positive for antiphospholipid antibodies.

History, examination and investigations
History
After focusing on the specific complaints of the patient referable to the joints and/or spine, one should then look at general aspects of the history that may provide further clues to the diagnosis. This aspect of the history taking is critically dependent on an adequate knowledge of the various diseases that one is diagnosing. This list cannot be all-inclusive, but the major points are outlined in Fig. 9.

Fig. 9 Generic aspects
of the history

Generic aspects of the history
Systemic features • anorexia • weight loss • fever **Organ dysfunction** • change in pattern/symptoms micturition • change/alteration in bowel habits • skin manifestations • cough, haemoptysis **Social history** • smoking and alcohol history • exercise • menopause **Family history** • seronegative arthritis • psoriasis, inflammatory bowel disease • uveitis • rheumatoid arthritis

❝ The history of anorexia, weight loss or fever should always be sought, particularly when there is an acute onset of spinal disease ❞

Systemic features

The history of anorexia, weight loss or fever should always be sought, particularly when there is an acute onset of spinal disease. Anorexia and weight loss may suggest a malignancy or inflammatory bowel disease. Fever may suggest an infection either in the spine or in the joint. These are important sentinel aspects of the history.

Organ dysfunction

The history should include appropriate direct questioning to elicit possible organ dysfunction. Changes in the pattern and frequency of micturition and whether there are symptoms on micturition such as burning or discomfort could be a clue to sexually transmitted disease and the diagnosis of a reactive arthritis. Changes or alterations in bowel habits with diarrhoea and looseness of motions may have been going on for some time in a patient who has unknown inflammatory bowel disease. Acute intestinal infection can present in this manner and may be followed 2 weeks later by development of reactive arthritis. Skin manifestations such as psoriasis are very important in making the correct diagnosis. Finally, symptoms directly referable to an organ dysfunction such as a cough or haemoptysis from the lung, haematuria from the kidney or sphincter disturbance should alert one to the possibility of other diseases contributing to the patient's symptoms.

Social history

Social history is extremely important. Smoking and alcohol consumption are associated with women who develop osteoporotic vertebral collapse. Lack of exercise in a woman may contribute to the development of osteoporosis while work habits may predispose an individual to OA of a specific joint or joint groups, for example, of the hip in farmers. The date of onset of the menopause is obviously critical in establishing whether there is a possibility of postmenopausal osteoporosis.

Family history

Although the family history is important in reaching a diagnosis, most musculoskeletal diseases have a very low familial component. The one exception is ankylosing spondylitis where a family history is frequently obtained. Nevertheless, a history should be taken as to whether there is seronegative arthritis, psoriasis, inflammatory bowel disease and uveitis in family members as any of these can be found in patients who present with seronegative arthritis with or without spondylitis. Finally, family history of RA should be obtained although multi-case RA families are rare.

Principles of clinical examination

In discussing the principles of clinical examination, the scheme of symptom presentation for arthritis, spinal disease and CTD should be borne in mind.

Joint examination

Joints have their own particular range of motion and patients should be asked to actively move the joints being complained of through their normal range of movement. Subsequent passive examination may elicit whether the failure to voluntarily move the joint is due to a joint problem itself or perhaps a neurological complication. The size of the joint and whether there is an effusion should be established by appropriate clinical tests. Some joints are easier to examine, from the point of view of an effusion, than others: it is easier to detect a knee effusion than an effusion in the shoulder. Whether a joint is tender on palpation or movement is an important clinical finding. The colour of the overlying skin should also be noted. An erythematous skin over a joint with exquisite tenderness would suggest crystal arthritis. As many joints of the patient as possible should be examined as the most important distinction is between a monoarthritis, oligoarthritis and a polyarthritis. From this simple distinction, the whole diagnostic panorama opens up.

> *"The date of onset of the menopause is obviously critical in establishing whether there is a possibility of postmenopausal osteoporosis."*

> *"As many joints of the patient as possible should be examined as the most important distinction is between a monoarthritis, oligoarthritis and a polyarthritis"*

Spinal examination

Examination of the cervical and lumbar spine should follow the same principles as that of the joints. Patients should be asked to move the neck and lumbar spine voluntarily so that the degree of movement can be ascertained. This should then be repeated passively so that the examiner can gauge the degree of restriction of movement. Swellings and other deformities should be sought and palpation and percussion should be used to elicit any tender areas. A neurological examination is indicated particularly when there are radicular symptoms.

Connective tissue diseases

Since CTDs can present in large and diverse forms and may involve virtually any organ system of the body, the summary of the clinical examination is difficult. Relevant parts of the clinical examination suggested by the history should be undertaken as thoroughly as possible.

Investigations

The investigations carried out in primary care depend on the diagnostic algorithm

The investigations carried out will depend critically on the history and clinical findings. One of the most appealing aspects of musculoskeletal disorders is that the vast majority can be diagnosed with a high degree of certainty on the basis of these two clinical skills. Most of the rest can be diagnosed with relatively simple investigations, most of which are available to GPs. Rarer or more complex conditions will require further investigation by a rheumatologist who has access to specialist investigations as well as specialist imaging technology.

Tests should be based on a diagnostic algorithm

The investigations carried out in primary care depend on the diagnostic algorithm. This can be simplified as follows:
- whether there is monoarthritis or polyarthritis and whether the condition is acute or chronic,
- whether there is acute or chronic pain in the spine,
- suggestions of a CTD,
- evidence of systemic features compatible with polymyalgia rheumatica (PMR) or fever or weight loss,
- evidence of vasculitic involvement, which usually means giant cell arteritis (GCA) in the primary care setting.

Tests should be used to distinguish between the differential diagnoses

Investigations can be used to distinguish between different members of these various groupings

Investigations can be used to distinguish between different members of these various groupings. A convenient approach is as follows:
- Routine dipstick examination of the urine may reveal protein or

blood and may therefore suggest a CTD involving the kidneys.

- Elevated erythrocyte sedimentation rate (ESR) or C-reactive protein (CRP) will indicate the presence of inflammation, infection or neoplasia. These simple investigations immediately distinguish between inflammatory arthritis and non-inflammatory arthritis, and will include PMR and GCA, malignant disease and the CTDs.
- Biochemical investigations will indicate renal insufficiency, bone disease (elevation of alkaline phosphatase) and gout (elevated uric acid).
- Elevated creatinine kinase indicates polymyositis or dermatomyositis.
- Haematological investigation may reveal the normochromic normocytic anaemia of chronic inflammation, which may be present in RA or in malignancy.
  - Thrombocytopenia may be present in SLE.
  - Neutropenia in Felty's syndrome is a complication of RA.
  - Leucopenia is a manifestation of SLE.
  - A positive RF is found in RA and in primary SjS. RF positivity in early RA may be low. Beware of a positive latex screening test: this sensitive test should not be considered relevant in terms of a diagnosis except if a more specific test, such as the Rose-Waaler agglutination test, is positive.
  - A positive anti-nuclear antibody (ANA) opens the possibility of SLE or other CTD. A positive ANA test should alert the laboratory to carry out more specific tests for SLE. The classic autoantibodies in SLE are antibodies to double-stranded DNA.
  - A number of antigens that are extracted from the nuclei of cells – extractable nuclear antigens (ENA) – are diagnostic of other CTDs such as scleroderma and polymyositis. Their exact nomenclature is not relevant here. The most common antibodies to ENA are Ro/La, which are found in primary SjS. If such autoantibodies are present, a telephone call to the rheumatologist will lead to an explanation of their relevance and significance. Once positive, autoantibody tests remain positive and should not be repeated unless there is good reason.
- Serum immunoglobulin and electrophoresis for multiple myeloma are appropriate in a patient with systemic features or features suggestive of PMR.

"Beware of a positive latex screening test: this sensitive test should not be considered relevant in terms of a diagnosis except if a more specific test, such as the Rose–Waaler agglutination test, is positive"

"A positive ANA test should alert the laboratory to carry out more specific tests for SLE"

"Once positive, autoantibody tests remain positive and should not be repeated unless there is good reason"

Radiological examination

As a rule, the imaging technique available in primary care is plain radiography. The choice of site to be X-rayed will be dictated by the patient's symptoms. Some special points include:

- If a diagnosis of RA is being contemplated, plain radiographs of the hands and the feet should be obtained. The first erosions in

66 *The first
erosions in
rheumatoid
arthritis occur
in the feet. The
diagnosis of
rheumatoid
arthritis
depends
critically on the
symmetrical
involvement of
several joint
groups* 99

RA occur in the feet. The diagnosis of RA depends critically on the symmetrical involvement of several joint groups.

- If ankylosing spondylosis is being contemplated, radiological examination of the sacroiliac joints should be complemented with an anteroposterior and lateral view of the thoracolumbar region of the spine, as this is the area where syndesmophytes first appear.
- Acute arthritis may be due to gout: X-ray, usually of the feet, may show the typical punched-out erosions or pseudogout that will be demonstrated as chondrocalcinosis.

General comments

The performance of these basic investigations will speed the consultation process if the patient is to be referred to a rheumatologist. One of the advantages of electronic booking systems, as discussed in the final chapter, is that the relevant investigations can be flagged up during the booking procedure and can be carried out and be available before the consultation itself.

Back pain

66 *The performance
of these basic
investigations
will speed the
consultation
process if the
patient is to be
referred to a
rheumatologist* 99

Dealing with back pain efficiently is a practical necessity in primary care because it is so commonplace. Few patients will be referred to back pain clinics or secondary care and rarely will surgery be indicated. Look for red flags at the first consultation and also be aware of potential psychological factors (yellow flags).

Presentation of back pain in primary care

- pain in the back,
- pain radiating into the legs,
- "stiffness" in the back,
- lumbago,
- back locking.

Most will be simple backache as defined by the RCGP Back Pain Guidelines:

- patient aged 20–55 years,
- lumbosacral region, buttocks and thighs affected,
- pain "mechanical" in nature, i.e., varies with level of physical activity, time of day, and day to day,
- patient well,
- prognosis good: 90% recover from an acute attack within 6 weeks.

Problems of simple backache

At least 10% of patients with simple backache will have psychosocial problems that may delay recovery. These problems can be aggravated by employers requiring patients to be fully fit before returning to work. It is important that patients remain at work when practical, but this is not possible when employers demand that workers are 100% fit. Try to anticipate and discuss potential problems early in the consultation process. Be pro-active with patients who return for an appointment sooner than planned or who make further appointments with partners or other health staff.

Psychosocial assessments
* Consider attitudes and beliefs about:
  - back pain,
  - fear avoidance,
  - activity and work responsibility,
  - rehabilitation,
  - family (especially partners) attitudes and beliefs.
* Psychological distress and depressive symptoms.
* Illness behaviour/non-health problems causing time off work, etc:
  - patient using back pain as a way of improving/obtaining social housing, or
  - patients using back pain as a means of obtaining social security benefits.
* Work
  - physical demands of work,
  - job satisfaction,
  - other health problems causing absence from work,
  - employers attitudes.

Nerve root pain
A very small percentage of patients will have nerve root pain. Symptoms are:
* unilateral leg pain worse than low back pain (or back pain may be absent),
* pain generally radiates below the knee to the foot or toe,
* numbness or paraesthesia in the same distribution,
* nerve irritation signs, i.e., reduced straight leg raising and production of leg pain (Fig. 10),
* motor, sensory or reflex changes limited to one nerve root.

Prognosis is reasonable; 50% of patients recover from this acute attack in 6 weeks, although it can last 6 months.

In primary care, triage should be routine. Listening and looking for red flags, cauda equina syndromes and inflammatory disorders should become second nature. Time spent here pays dividends. Examination will confirm suspicions but will rarely produce a "new" diagnosis.

***A very small percentage of patients will have nerve root pain**

23

Fig. 10 Examination for pain in the back: supine position. Reprinted from Standards in Rheumatology: A Suggested Management Plan for Some Common Conditions in Rheumatology, The Medicine Group 1987.

a When supine, the nerve roots (L4, L5 and S1) are slack

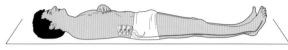

b Straight leg raising is limited by the tension of the root over the prolapsed disc

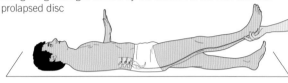

c Tension is increased by dorsiflexion of the foot

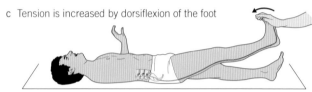

d Root tension is relieved by flexion at the knee

e With the knee extended, the root tightens over the prolapsed disc causing pain which radiates to the back

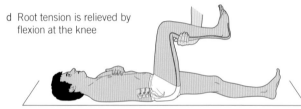

f Pressure over the centre of the popliteal fossa pulls on the posterior tibial nerve which is "bow stringing" across the fossa causing local pain and radiation to the back

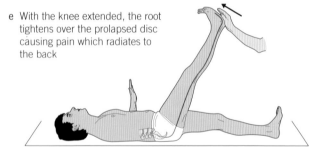

Red flags for possible serious events
* age of onset < 20 or > 55 years,
* severe trauma,
* progressive and constant pain,
* thoracic pain,
* history of carcinoma,
* systemic steroids,
* drug abuse, HIV, TB,
* systemically unwell,
* weight loss,
* persisting, severe restriction of lumbar flexion,
* structural deformity,
* symptoms worse in the mornings,
* nocturnal pain.

Cauda equina syndrome/severe neurological problem
Look for the following:
* widespread neurology,
* difficulty with micturition,
* saddle anaesthesia: does it feel normal when wiping or drying the bottom,
* sensory level.

Inflammatory disorders
The back conditions that rheumatologists, and patients, *do not* want missed and that *do* need referral to secondary care are the inflammatory disorders. These are not easy to identify in the early stages when symptoms are mild, e.g., a woman may have a slightly stiff back in the morning and have some difficulty in washing her face, or sitting for long periods may be uncomfortable and a student may prefer to stand at the back of the lecture hall rather than sit.

> *The back conditions that rheumatologists, and patients, do not want missed and that do need referral to secondary care are the inflammatory disorders*

Classic symptoms of ankylosing spondylitis and related disorders
* gradual onset before the age of 40 years,
* marked morning stiffness,
* nocturnal awakening in the small hours,
* persisting limitation of spinal movements,
* peripheral joint involvement (not always),
* iritis, skin rashes (psoriasis), colitis, urethral discharge,
* positive family history.

What clinical examination is necessary?

"A patient should be fully examined, preferably on the first or second visit, but definitely on the first visit if the history suggests red flags"

A patient should be fully examined, preferably on the first or second visit, but definitely on the first visit if the history suggests red flags. Patient standing:

- gait and posture of the patient entering the surgery,
- time and ease of undressing,
- consistency of movement restriction,
- is the spine straight?
- pelvic alignment,
- movements: compare the left and right sides in:
  - flexion,
  - extension,
  - rotation (also with patient sitting); beware of rigid or stiff spine.
- axial compression: push down on the patient's head; this should not be painful but it is likely to be positive if yellow flags are present,
- standing on toes tests calf muscles (innervated by S1 nerve root).

Patient lying on their back (Fig. 10)

- straight leg raise and sciatic nerve stretch,
- hip movements,
- sacroiliac joint springing (unreliable),
- reflexes,
- power in legs,
- sensation (remember saddle anaesthesia),
- abdominal examination.

Patient prone (Fig. 11)

- femoral nerve stretch test,
- local tenderness in spine or pelvis.

"Worries concerning chronicity should arise in the first or second consultation"

Worries concerning chronicity should arise in the first or second consultation.

Risk factors for chronicity

- previous history and disproportionate illness behaviour,
- absence from work and low job satisfaction,
- radiation of pain and reduced raising of the straight leg,
- poor physical fitness and poor body image,
- heavy smoker,
- depressive symptoms/psychological distress/personal problems,
- insurance claims/compensation proceedings/housing problems.

Practical management of low back pain

When time is at a premium, consider a two-consultation approach.

a Patient prone; nerve roots (L2, L3 and L4) slack

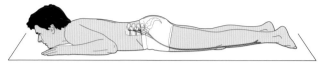

Fig. 11 Examination for pain in the back: prone position. Reprinted from Standards in Rheumatology: A Suggested Management Plan for Some Common Conditions in Rheumatology, The Medicine Group 1987.

b The femoral root is tightened by flexion of the knee. Pain may radiate from the back

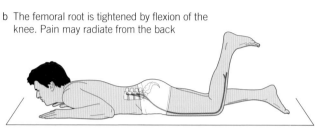

c If the previous movement does not cause pain, the femoral roots are further tensed by extension of the hip

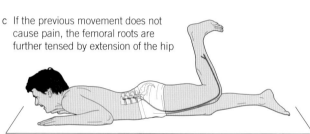

First consultation

*   Take a history and examine the patient (a brief examination is still worthwhile).
*   Exclude red flags; treat or refer as necessary.
*   Give appropriate education and advice regarding rest, posture, exercise and daily living.
*   Give analgesics and non-steroidal anti-inflammatory drugs (NSAIDs)/cyclo-oxygenase 2 inhibitors (Cox-2s) as appropriate.
*   Arrange physiotherapy/manipulation, if appropriate.

Second consultation

*   Often necessary if still experiencing pain at 2–3 weeks.
*   Full examination, if not done previously.
*   Assess psychosocial areas (yellow flags).
*   Review analgesia; consider muscle relaxants and antidepressants.
*   Remember nerve root pain has a prolonged course.

Only a very small number of painful backs warrant X-ray investigation. Ask the question, "Will it change the management?"

❝ Only a very small number of painful backs warrant X-ray investigation. Ask the question, 'Will it change the management?' ❞

Neck pain

> *Primary care must apply the same principles of triage to the neck as for lower back pain. If these principles are applied, patients can be managed with confidence*

Most patients with neck pain have mechanical neck pain (equivalent to mechanical lower back pain) and should be treated similarly for each episode. As with low back pain, neck pain may be an acute attack or a chronic problem. The latter may have intermittent exacerbation.

Mechanical pain means pain related to movement and activities and which is relieved by rest. Excessive local muscular activity may cause patients to describe discomfort in the neck, trapezius and supraspinatus muscles and to have tender points in the same muscles.

Primary care must apply the same principles of triage to the neck as for lower back pain. If these principles are applied, patients can be managed with confidence.

Nerve root pain equivalent to sciatic pain

Pain radiates to the shoulder and upper arm, or further down the arm, even to the thumb and fingers, and some reflexes may be diminished. Affected areas and reflexes will help distinguish which root is irritated (affected). The most common roots involved are C5, C6 and C7 (Fig. 12).

It is important to realise that this problem is very similar to sciatic or femoral nerve irritation. Management is the same and recovery is similarly protracted. X-rays are rarely helpful. Conventional views are useless but oblique views may show encroachment into the foramina by osteophytes. The report is usually on the lines of cervical spondylosis at C5/C6". In most cases, it is important to treat the patient's symptoms,

Fig. 12 Segmental distribution of symptoms,
http://www.arc.org.uk/about_arth/med_reports/series4/ip/6507/6507.htm

Segmental distribution of symptoms	
C5 root	Pain radiates to the shoulder and the anterior upper arm, along with weakness of the deltoid muscle, diminished biceps and pectoral reflex and sensory changes over the deltoid (the regimental badge area).
C6 root	Pain radiates into the lateral arm and the dorsal aspect of the forearm with weakness in the biceps muscle. Sensory changes occur in the thumb and the dorsal surface of the hand. The biceps and brachioradialis reflexes may be diminished or absent.
C7 root	Pain affects the forearm and middle and ring fingers. Weakness of the triceps and the extensors of the wrist and fingers may occur. Sensory deficit if present is in the index and middle fingers. The triceps reflex may be reduced.
C8 root	Pain occurs in the medial aspect of the arm and forearm with weakness in the intrinsic muscles of the hand. Paraesthesia may arise in the ring and little fingers and along the medial side of the forearm. Arm reflexes are preserved.

not the X-ray. The patient will require reassurance, explanation, physio-therapy and pain relief. Reassessment is needed to ascertain that there is no progression, which is uncommon but must always be considered.

Progressive neurological deficit

This usually develops insidiously, either stepwise or gradually. The initial phase may be followed by a stable period often lasting years.

> *Progressive neurological deficit usually develops insidiously, either stepwise or gradually*

What does the patient notice?

Upper limbs:
- impaired coordination of hands,
- difficulty fastening buttons,
- weakness and wasting of hand muscles,
- grip may be slow and stiff.

Lower limbs:
- gait disturbance from spasticity and weakness.

What signs are important?

- Exaggerated reflexes below the level of the lesion.
- Plantar response may be extensor, also clonus elicited.
- Beware: sensory disturbance may be minimal and only in the upper limb.
- 80% of patients have loss of vibration sensation in the legs and impaired joint position.
- Only 50% have bladder sphincter symptoms (urgency).
- A central cord syndrome usually produces weak arms and hands but spares lower limb function.

What is the differential diagnosis for progressive neurological deficit?

- Around 12% of patients with the above problems (features rarely seen in primary care) will have even rarer conditions such as:
  - intraspinal tumours,
  - syringomyelia,
  - Arnold-Chiari malformations.
- Other conditions causing secondary care difficulties are:
  - amyotrophic lateral sclerosis,
  - chronic severe RA that leads to cervical instability and progressive neurological deficit.

Who warrants surgical referral?

In primary care, this means "Who should be referred?" NOT "Who requires surgery?".

29

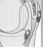
> ❝Urgent referral is reserved for patients with severe neurological deficit especially in the case of rapid or relatively rapid progression ❞

> ❝Patients who have neck pain plus nerve root symptoms should also be managed conservatively (c.f., back pain management) ❞

- Patients with persistent nerve root pain who do not respond to conservative management and intensive physiotherapy.
- Intermittent arm symptoms (like intermittent sciatica), or symptoms brought on by lifting or by carrying shopping, usually resolve though recovery is prolonged. Patients warrant referral if the symptoms become constant.
- Urgent referral is reserved for patients with severe neurological deficit especially in the case of rapid or relatively rapid progression.

Patients with "simple" or uncomplicated neck pain (cervical spondylosis on X-ray) should NOT be referred. These patients have localized neck pain with muscle overactivity of the cervical spine and shoulder girdles. They do not have nerve root pain. As in low back pain, surgery without neurological complications is unproven and patients are best managed conservatively. Patients who have neck pain plus nerve root symptoms should also be managed conservatively (c.f., back pain management).

Examination – an aide mémoire

Look: check cervical and thoracic spines and shoulders, for swellings, deformity and posture.

Feel: this helps reassure the patient whilst checking for local tenderness over muscles and severe pain over bony areas. The latter may signify a serious problem.

Move: (Fig. 13). Remember:

- Neck movements decrease with age (especially lateral flexion).
- Pain is exacerbated by lateral flexion away from the affected side as this stretches the affected root.

Neurology:

- The history will suggest root problems that need to be recorded in the case notes. Fig. 12 may help diagnose which root is affected.
- Remember to check lower limbs, especially plantars.

Investigations

- Cervical spine X-rays are rarely necessary and should be reserved for patients who have root symptoms that are not responding to conservative treatment. Unfortunately, this is not always practical in the clinical/psychosocial setting. If an X-ray is necessary, ask for an oblique view that will exclude encroachment into the foramina by osteophytes.
- Other specialist investigations should be the domain of secondary care.

Fig. 13 Examination of the neck: movements.
Reprinted from Klippel JH, et al. Primary Care Rheumatology, Mosby 1999. (opposite page)

Cervical spine		
Right rotation	**Left rotation**	**Flexion**

	Right rotation		Left rotation		Flexion
Manoeuvre	Turn head to right	Manoeuvre	Turn head to left	Manoeuvre	Flex neck forward
Assessment	Estimate angle	Assessment	Estimate angle	Assessment	Estimate angle
Normal angle	60–90° diminishing with age	Normal angle	60–90° diminishing with age	Normal angle	60–90° diminishing with age
Active/passive	Active	Active/passive	Active	Active/passive	Active

Right rotation	Left rotation	Flexion
The patient sits comfortably on the edge of the examining table with the legs hanging free, facing the examiner. The patient is asked to turn his/her head to the right as far as possible. The examiner gently guides the patient's jaw to ensure that the maximum range is achieved, and then estimates the angle.	The patient sits comfortably on the edge of the examining table with the legs hanging free, facing the examiner. The patient is asked to turn his/her head to the left as far as possible. The examiner gently guides the patient's jaw to ensure that maximum range is achieved, and then estimates the angle.	The patient sits comfortably on the edge of the examining table with the legs hanging free, facing the examiner. The patient is asked to bend his/her head forward as far as possible. The examiner gently guides the patient's head to ensure that the maximum range is achieved, and then estimates the angle.

Extension	**Right lateral flexion**	**Left lateral flexion**

	Extension		Right lateral flexion		Left lateral flexion
Manoeuvre	--	Manoeuvre	Flex neck to right	Manoeuvre	Flex neck to left
Assessment	Estimate angle	Assessment	Estimate angle	Assessment	Estimate angle
Normal angle	60–90° diminishing with age	Normal angle	60–90° diminishing with age	Normal angle	60–90° diminishing with age
Active/passive	Active	Active/passive	Active	Active/passive	Active

Extension	Right lateral flexion	Left lateral flexion
The patient sits comfortably on the edge of the examining table with the legs hanging free, facing the examiner. The patient is asked to look up as far as he/she can. The examiner gently guides the patient's jaw to ensure that the maximum range is achieved, and then estimates the angle.	The patient sits comfortably on the edge of the examining table with the legs hanging free, facing the examiner. The patient is asked to angle his/her head to the right to try to touch his/her ear with his/her shoulder. The examiner gently guides the patient's head to ensure that the maximum range is achieved, and then estimates the angle.	The patient sits comfortably on the edge of the examining table with the legs hanging free, facing the examiner. The patient is asked to angle his/her head to the left to try to touch his/her ear with his/her shoulder. The examiner gently guides the patient's head to ensure that the maximum range is achieved, and then estimates the angle.

31

Management of neck pain

This should be similar to back pain management.

Pain management approach (conservative)

Based in primary care:
- Relieve symptoms.
- Reassure concerning symptoms: pain, though unpleasant, is safe; moving the head will not do any damage nor will the head fall off!
- Encourage to remain active, which includes working despite the pain.
- Use analgesics (NSAIDs/Cox-2s and muscle relaxants) appropriately to encourage active mobilization.
- Where necessary, refer to physiotherapy (mandatory for nerve root symptoms).
- Soft collars, like back supports, should rarely be used. Use of rigid neck collars (for severe root symptoms) should be restricted to secondary care.

Knee pain

Knee pain is a common problem, bringing patients of all ages to the primary care team (see also Musculoskeletal problems in children and teenagers and the active elderly, page 85).

Examination

Examination for effusion

The patellar tap test is positive with a moderate effusion, usually ≥ 20mL of fluid.

Two methods demonstrate an effusion of the knee, both with the patient lying prone. The *patellar tap test* is positive with a moderate effusion, usually ≥ 20mL of fluid.
- With the non-dominant hand, squash fluid from the suprapatellar pouch to behind the patella. Keep this hand over the pouch.
- Using the thumb or a finger of the dominant hand, press sharply over the centre of the patella, as if playing a piano note.
- The patella will move between the finger and the femur, called balloting.

The *swipe* (or bulge or cross-fluctuation) *test* is useful for detecting small effusions of 5–10mL.
- Stabilize the patella with a thumb.
- Stroke downwards on the medial compartment of the knee. This moves all the fluid into the lateral compartment.
- Keeping the patella stabilized, swipe the lateral compartment with the back of the hand and look for a bulge of the medial compartment.

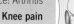

Examination for anterior knee pain

- With the patient lying flat on the couch, use the index finger and thumb of the non-dominant hand to stabilize the patella over the femur.
- Using the dominant index finger, press down in a localized, grinding, rotational motion over each of the four quadrants of the patella. Ask the patient if this action produces pain.
- In most patients with patellofemoral problems, pain will be elicited in the upper and sometimes the lower lateral quadrants of the patella.
- In the severest cases, all four quadrants are painful.

This test has replaced compression of the patella onto the femoral condyle, where the patient is asked to contract the quadriceps, as this may produce severe pain.

Testing collateral ligaments

- With the patient supine on the couch, flex the knee to about 30°. This relaxes the posterior capsule and the posterior cruciate ligament.
- Grip the ankle with one hand and place the other hand at the joint line behind the knee. Exert a force laterally at the ankle to check for medial stability.
- For lateral stability, exert a medial force at the ankle.

Some practitioners may need to change hands to undertake these stability tests.

There are two tests for anterior cruciate ligament (ACL) integrity.

In *Lachman's test* for anterior cruciate laxity:

- Flex the knee to 20–30°, possibly over the examiner's own leg or over a hard pillow. This relaxes the capsule and the posterior cruciate ligament.
- Grasp the femur with the non-dominant hand and the tibia with the dominant hand.
- Try to pull the tibia forward while keeping the femur stable.
- If the cruciate ligament is damaged, the tibia will have greater movement compared to the good leg.

There are two draw tests. The *anterior draw test* assesses excessive movement of the tibia in relation to the femur:

- With the patient lying flat on the couch, flex the hip to 45° and the knee to 90°.
- Place the hands behind the tibia and pull forwards.
- Too much movement suggests instability and even ACL rupture. Remember to compare with the good knee.

For the *posterior draw test*:

- Position as for the anterior draw test except that the tibia is pushed posteriorly.

> **❝The** anterior draw test *assesses excessive movement of the tibia in relation to the femur* **❞**

- Too much movement suggests a ruptured posterior cruciate ligament.
- This may be suspected on inspection by placing both knees at 90° and comparing both profiles. If there is loss of the posterior cruciate, the tibial profile will appear flatter and as if it has slipped posteriorly compared to the normal knee.

Fig. 14 Signs and symptoms of meniscal problems

Signs and symptoms of meniscal problems

- locking
- limited extension
- joint line tenderness, which may be present at different degrees of flexion
- grating of the knee on movement rather than crepitus
- effusion which may be acute or recurrent
- quadriceps wasting, which may be more severe than expected

Fig. 15 Common causes of knee pain relevant to age

Age	Joint causes	Around the joint	Referred pain to the knee
10–18 years	Osteochondritis dissecans Torn meniscus Anterior knee pain • Hypermobility • Patellar malalignment	Osgood-Schlatter's syndrome Sinding-Larsen-Johansson syndrome Osteomyelitis Tumours	Slipped upper femoral epiphysis
Early adulthood (18–30 years)	Torn meniscus Anterior knee pain • Hypermobility • Instability Inflammatory conditions	Overuse syndromes Bursitis Sports injuries to tendons	
Adulthood (30–50 years)	Meniscal tears Anterior knee pain • Hypermobility Early degeneration • Previous injury • Previous meniscectomy Inflammatory arthropathies	Bursitis Tendonitis Sports injuries to tendons Baker's cyst	Referred pain from hip conditions (pain to front of thigh and knee)
Older adulthood (> 50 years)	OA Inflammatory arthropathies Hypermobility	Bursitis Tendonitis Sports injuries Baker's cyst	Referred pain from osteoarthritis of the hip

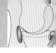

It is sensible to perform both draw tests and Lachman's test if a cruciate problem is suspected. The definitive investigation is magnetic resonance imaging (MRI).

Examination for meniscal tears

These are always inconclusive in non-specialist hands and rarely conclusive when performed by an expert. The key to meniscal problems is the history and signs and symptoms (Fig. 14).

Sports problems of the knee in adolescence and other age groups

Fig. 15 lists common causes of knee pain relevant to age.

Osteochondritis dissecans

This is probably a fatigue or an over-use type of injury, typically affecting the medial femoral condyle. It is quite different from a meniscal injury, where there is a loss of knee extension of 5–10°. Be suspicious in patients who have:

- an aching knee,
- an effusion,
- a loose fragment within the knee joint, usually seen on X-ray, or
- knee locking that can be reversed by a shake of the knee.

Osgood-Schlatter's (tibial end) and Sinding-Larsen-Johannson (patella end) syndromes

These traction osteochondroses affect a specific end of the patella tendon and cause localized swelling and tenderness. Treatment is conservative and includes decreasing overactivity and maintaining the patient's fitness by changing the exercise remit, for example, swimming or cycling. Immobilization and surgery are desperate resorts.

These syndromes are probably biomechanical in origin and occur in very active sports persons who are growing rapidly. There is a mismatch of bone length and muscle length. Treatment probably "buys time" for this mismatch to resolve.

Other scenarios suggested by a good case history

A patient of any age who complains of the knee "giving way" or "letting down" requires further questioning to elucidate the following problems:

- pain on turning = meniscus tear,
- gives way on turning = ACL problem,
- anterior knee pain (when going down stairs or walking down hill) = patellofemoral problem,
- transient locking and sharp twinges of pain = loose body.

> **It is sensible to perform both draw tests and Lachman's test if a cruciate problem is suspected**

> **A patient of any age who complains of the knee "giving way" or "letting down" requires further questioning**

35

Medial meniscus injuries

These are common, especially in footballers. They occur when the foot is fixed and a rotational force is applied. The case history is very important and classically includes sudden pain plus a click. There may also be a history of an effusion, which may have resolved but may recur with each painful episode. The patient may be unable to fully extend the knee and will have lost quadriceps bulk (Fig. 14).

Anterior knee pain in athletically active adolescents/patellar malalignment (chondromalacia patella)

The most common problem underlying this symptom is hypermobility causing joints to overflex and -extend. The muscles protect the joints (major shock absorbers) and restrain the joint from overextension or overflexion. A simple concept is that at times of rapid growth, muscles and bones do not grow at exactly the same rate. Girls present at approximately 13 years complaining of knee pain, boys usually a few years later. Remember to check for hypermobility in all patients presenting with joint or muscle problems (pages 83–85). There may be enough joint laxity to cause subluxation of the patella. Treatment is quadriceps exercises and, rarely, patella release. Patients should be advised to wear trainers, no matter what the occasion. If knee pain is very severe, it is worthwhile taking an old pair of trainers, cutting the heels off and replacing them with thin, rubber ones that can be bought in most supermarkets (glue them on). This lowers the heel and will stop overextension of the knee and should give good pain relief.

Early adulthood knee problems

Anterior knee pain (biomechanical problem)

This is quite common and usually presents with hypermobile joints in patients who previously had quality quadriceps. Because of a change in circumstances (work, etc), they allowed the quadriceps to decay but have now returned to some form of exercise, although they no longer have good protectors. Treat as above and see section on hypermobility (pages 83–85).

Bursitis around the knee

Bursae are fibrous sacs that act as lubricating structures, reducing friction at bony prominences (Fig. 16). The suprapatellar bursa communicates directly with the knee joint.

❝ Bursae are fibrous sacs that act as lubricating structures, reducing friction at bony prominences ❞

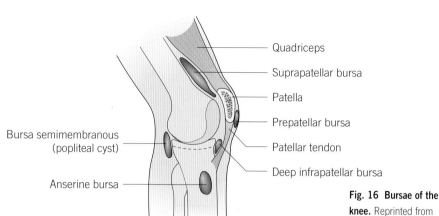

Labels:
- Quadriceps
- Suprapatellar bursa
- Patella
- Prepatellar bursa
- Patellar tendon
- Deep infrapatellar bursa
- Bursa semimembranous (popliteal cyst)
- Anserine bursa

Fig. 16 Bursae of the knee. Reprinted from Hosie GAC and Field M, Shared Care for Rheumatology, Martin Dunitz 2002.

Sports injuries
Haemarthrosis
This develops within an hour or so of the injury occurring, whereas a synovial fluid effusion develops overnight. The joint feels tight and is tense. Usual causes include:

- ACL rupture,
- peripheral tear of the medial meniscus,
- patella dislocation.

Recurrent small knee effusions
These are rarely painless but the pain may be fleeting and largely discounted by the patient. Causes include:
- trapping of the joint capsule in a hypermobile joint,
- minimal displacement of the patella, usually in a hypermobile joint,
- an old injury to a meniscus,
- extension of a meniscus tear,
- minimal locking or unlocking of a torn meniscus.

An effusion in a sports person requires drainage, otherwise there is extensive loss of quadriceps bulk and power. Ultrasound or MRI is more likely to be of value than plain X-ray and should be requested at recurrence or sooner, depending on individual circumstances.

Medial collateral ligament injury
Classically a skiing injury (catching an edge), caused by an external rotation force or, in contact sports, a blow to the side of the knee.

An effusion in a sports person requires drainage, otherwise there is extensive loss of quadriceps bulk and power

Anterior cruciate ligament injury

This common injury is easily missed. The history classically includes a flexion/rotation stress when descending from a jump. Examination shows haemarthrosis, i.e., traumatic synovitis with restriction of passive flexion/extension. Haemarthrosis is usually accompanied by painful movements and is a warm, tense, more boggy effusion than synovial effusion.

Posterior cruciate ligament injury

This is more common in road traffic accidents (knee against the dashboard) and is less likely to be caused by sports. If caused by a sports injury, the patient rarely returns to contact sports. Repairs are not successful compared with ACL repairs.

Lateral collateral ligament injury

This varus stress is uncommon. When it does occur, the ACL is usually damaged too.

Inflammatory conditions

These are treated in secondary care (RA chapter, page 90).

Adulthood 30–50 years
Early degeneration

Injuries to the ACL or menisci or surgery on the menisci may lead to early osteoarthritic changes, certainly on X-ray and often clinically. Clinical signs are pain, loss of some function and change in shape (squaring of the joint).

Osteoarthritis

See OA chapter, pages 67–73.

Referred pain at all ages

Hip pain can be referred to the knee *but* knee pain is not referred to the hip. Referred hip pain tends to give pain at the front of the knee and top of the thigh.

> **"** Hip pain can be referred to the knee but knee pain is not referred to the hip. Referred hip pain tends to give pain at the front of the knee and top of the thigh **"**

Hip pain
Signs and symptoms

Hip pain may present in three main areas: lateral hip, groin and buttock. It may also be referred to the front of the thighs. The most common causes of hip pain in primary care are:

- trochanteric bursitis,
- hip OA,
- femoral neck fractures,

- referred pain from the spine (and abdomen).

Less common causes include:
- buttock pain:
  - ischiogluteal bursitis,
  - sacroiliac joint disease,
- adductor tendonitis,
- osteonecrosis,
- meralgia paraesthetica,
- paget's disease (other bone diseases).

Trochanteric bursitis/subtrochanteric bursitis

Predisposing factors include:
- obesity,
- mechanical back pain,
- hip OA (treating the bursitis often gives patients relief from severe OA while awaiting surgery),
- bruising from falling,
- leg length discrepancies,
- sporting activities (even joggers).

This bursitis is more common in obese women than in men.
- Symptoms: deep ache, burning pain on lateral aspect of thigh, worse on exercise; patient may limp.
- Signs: tenderness over the greater trochanter (trochanteric bursitis) or below the greater trochanter at the level of the symphysis pubis (subtrochanteric bursitis) (Fig. 17).

❝ Tenderness over the greater trochanter (trochanteric bursitis) or below the greater trochanter at the level of the symphysis pubis (subtrochanteric bursitis) ❞

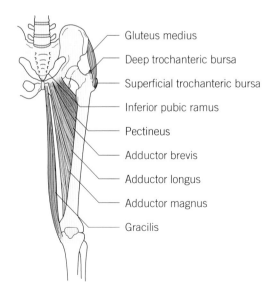

Gluteus medius

Deep trochanteric bursa

Superficial trochanteric bursa

Inferior pubic ramus

Pectineus

Adductor brevis

Adductor longus

Adductor magnus

Gracilis

Fig. 17 Inflammation of the superficial and deep trochanteric bursae and the upper leg muscles. Adapted from the University of Bath Diploma, Module 5 – Lower Limb.

Treatment for bursitis includes:

- Conservative treatments: rest, analgesics, NSAIDs/Cox-2s.
- If these fail, ultrasound may help.
- Preferred treatment is local anaesthetic plus steroid into the point of maximum tenderness.
- If the cause is hip OA, injections are sometimes required into both the deep and superficial bursae, repeated as necessary.

Examination of the hip

When the patient is supine (Fig. 18):

- Flex the hip to 90° and bend the knee to a right angle so the lower leg acts as a pointer.
- Rotate the leg away from the body; this moves/rotates the head of the femur internally. Normal rotation is 35°. Rotate the leg across the midline for external rotation of the femoral head, normally 45°.

Fig. 18 Internal rotation of the hip: supine.
Reprinted from Hosie G and Dickson J, Managing Osteoarthritis in Primary Care, Blackwell Science 2000.

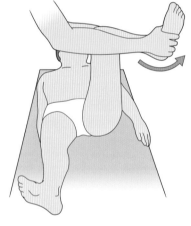

Fig. 19 Internal rotation of the hip: sitting.
Reprinted from Hosie G and Dickson J, Managing Osteoarthritis in Primary Care, Blackwell Science 2000.

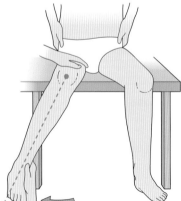

- Check flexion, normally 135°, by pushing the flexed knee up onto the chest wall.
- In hip disease, limitation of internal rotation usually occurs before limitation of hip flexion.

When the patient is sitting (Fig. 19), assess internal rotation (normally 35°):

- Patient sits on the end of a couch so that the legs don't touch the floor, with hands placed on hips.
- Stabilize the thigh with one hand; grip the lower end of the tibia and rotate the whole limb away from the body (laterally). Remember that the head of the femur will rotate internally.
- Watch the hands on the hips for the point when the hip begins to rise (limit of rotation).

Then assess external rotation (normally 45°):

- Rotate the whole of the limb across the body for external rotation of the femoral head.
- Watch the hands on the hips for the point when the hip begins to rise (limit of rotation).

If internal rotation of the hip is normal in a patient with possible hip OA, the patient does not require surgical referral and rarely an X-ray.

> *If internal rotation of the hip is normal in a patient with possible hip OA, the patient does not require surgical referral and rarely an X-ray*

Groin strain (adductor muscles)

- This is caused by turning quickly while weight bearing. It usually affects the adductor longus (Fig. 17), so pain is felt on the medial portion of the inferior pubic ramus, or on the inner side of the thigh.
- A tear is more likely in a footballer using the inside of his/her boot to kick a ball that cannot move (trapped under player's foot).
- Horse riders are prone to chronic adductor strain and may develop an enthesitis.
- Treatment is usually a mixture of quality physiotherapy, ultrasound and, sometimes, local anaesthetic and steroid injections. Surgery is rarely needed.

Ischial-gluteal bursitis

This gives a similar clinical pattern to chronic hamstring sprain:

- Discomfort in the back of the thigh and buttock.
- Pain on straight leg raising, but maximum tenderness over the ischial tuberosity compared to that with sciatic nerve root pain.
- Conservative treatment may be supplemented with injections of local anaesthetic and steroid.

Other less common problems

Osteonecrosis (avascular necrosis)

Consider this diagnosis in patients with hip pain of progressive severity, especially in people younger than 55 years. Causes are said to divide into:

- $1/3$ steroid usage,
- $1/3$ high alcohol intake, and
- $1/3$ idiopathic.

Meralgia paraesthetica

Symptoms include burning pain with numbness, paraesthesia and hyperalgesia over the lateral part of the thigh or in the groin. This syndrome is caused by compression of the lateral femoral cutaneous nerve of the thigh, either at the anterior superior iliac spine where the nerve runs under the lateral end of the inguinal ligament or where the nerve pierces the iliac fascia (the latter is "caught" on a table edge). Think of the diagnosis in a mother who carries her child on her hip or in people who wear tight clothes (e.g., jeans that have become wet). Give advice about clothes, etc, before considering local anaesthetic and steroid.

Paget's disease

- This is a localized disorder of bone remodelling.
- It is rare < 40 years of age and is more common in men than women.
- Most patients (70%) are asymptomatic.
- The major symptom is pain, which is often difficult to localize, even though the pain may be intense.
- Think of the diagnosis, check the serum alkaline phosphatase and consider an X-ray or ask secondary care for a bone scan.

Metastatic or primary bone tumours

❝Primary tumours of bone are rare❞

- Primary tumours of bone are rare.
- Be suspicious if the patient has constant pain in the bone, not relieved by rest and not affected by activity.
- Weight loss, tiredness and fevers are usually late systemic features.
- People with known primary tumours are always at risk of developing metastatic bone disease, commonly in the spine or hip. Be suspicious if the patient develops bone pain or fractures a bone. Classically, there is unremitting bone pain with some systemic features.
- Sometimes patients develop metastatic spread in the absence of a known primary, presenting similarly to a primary or because of a pathological fracture.

Shoulder pain

Pain is said to be acute if it has been present for less than 12 weeks and chronic if present for at least 12 weeks. The shoulder refers to the scapula, clavicle, humerus and associated ligaments, tendons, muscles and relevant soft tissues that are all in relationship with each other.

- 10% of the population will experience shoulder pain at least once in their life.
- It is the third most common cause of pain, after back and neck pain.
- 95% of all patients with shoulder pain are treated in primary care.
- 23% of new episodes resolve within 4 weeks.
- 44% resolve within 12 weeks.
- Risks of chronicity are similar to those for neck and low back pain.
- Yellow flags
  - personality traits,
  - coping style,
  - occupational factors.

Shoulder pain and its management

- Most shoulder pain is mechanical in origin and should be managed as *acute regional pain*.
- Always exclude red flags:
  - infection,
  - trauma, fracture, dislocation.
- History rarely helps as a diagnostic tool (similar to back and neck pain) but may alert one to the presence of red and yellow flags.
- Biological factors (age, female sex, history, response to repetitive tasks) may contribute to the development of shoulder pain.
- Psychosocial factors (yellow flags), such as job dissatisfaction, work demands, personality traits, home circumstances, may contribute to the onset and chronicity of shoulder pain.
- No clinical test is both reliable and valid for any specific diagnostic entity but examination of the patient enhances rapport and places the pain in context. Lack of a precise diagnosis does not preclude a satisfactory outcome.
- Rarely are X-rays or imaging necessary in primary care unless red flags are a distinct possibility.
- 50% of patients, treated conservatively, will recover in 6 months, rising to 60% in 12 months.
- Shoulder pain often recurs, even after an initial full recovery (similar to neck and back pain).
- Any management plan must consider biological and psychosocial risk factors.

"Pain is said to be acute if it has been present for less than 12 weeks and chronic if present for at least 12 weeks"

"No clinical test is both reliable and valid for any specific diagnostic entity but examination of the patient enhances rapport and places the pain in context"

Evidence for each intervention

- Topical and oral NSAIDs give moderate to small benefit for up to 4 weeks when compared to placebo.
- Subacromial injections of steroid may improve the shoulder pain at 4 weeks up to a maximum of 12 weeks.
- Acupuncture may help pain and function to a small degree in the short term.
- Physiotherapy may improve pain in the short term.

At present, there is no evidence to support or refute:

- efficacy or safety of extracorporeal shock wave therapy (ESWT),
- suprascapular nerve block,
- oral corticosteroids,
- surgery.

Practical shoulder examination

First, ask the patient where the pain is.

- Acromioclavicular joint problem: patient usually points to the pain over the acromioclavicular joint.
- Painful arc (also called rotator cuff, impingement, subacromial tendonitis): patient places the opposite hand over the upper part of the affected arm.

Fig. 20 Arcs of shoulder pain

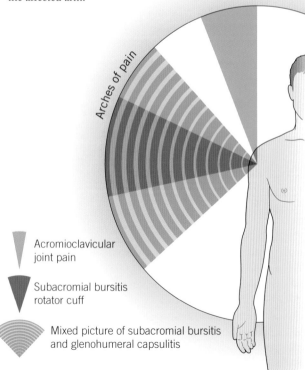

Arches of pain

Acromioclavicular joint pain

Subacromial bursitis rotator cuff

Mixed picture of subacromial bursitis and glenohumeral capsulitis

- Glenohumeral capsulitis: patient may say that it is difficult to localize the pain but that it is definitely in the shoulder.

With the patient standing:

- Begin with the arms by the sides. Ask the patient to raise the affected arm forwards, continue to above the head (making an arc with the hand), and describe any ensuing discomfort or pain.
- Ask the patient to repeat this arc with the palm facing forwards but the arm elevating sideways to above the head.
- Beginning with the arms by the side, ask the patient to "wash the back of the neck" with the affected arm, which uses external rotation. In glenohumeral capsulitis, this will be difficult or even impossible. Sometimes the patient compensates and will bring the hand and arm more medially up the inside of the body in order to wash and comb the hair.
- The clear picture of subacromial bursitis/rotator cuff tendonitis is common. If the patient has a pure rotator cuff problem, external rotation will be normal and their only complaint will be a painful arc.
- Some patients will have a mixed picture of rotator cuff tendonitis and glenohumeral capsulitis (some loss of external rotation) and so will have a much larger arc of pain or discomfort (Fig. 20).

❝ The clear picture of subacromial bursitis/rotator cuff tendonitis is common ❞

Practical management of shoulder pain

Each patient requires individualized treatment depending on the specific shoulder problem, the local circumstances and therapies available, and the experience and knowledge of the health practitioner. There has been a great increase in the knowledge base concerning shoulder pain.

- All treatment regimes must include either a self-managed exercise programme or physiotherapy sessions.
- At the end of 1 year, physiotherapy and steroid injections are equally effective.
- Steroid injections are more effective in the short term than physiotherapy.
- Chronic shoulder pain (> 2 years) causes considerable disability and can be compared to chronic back pain.

❝ All treatment regimes must include either a self-managed exercise programme or physiotherapy sessions ❞

Painful arc

This is also called rotator cuff tendonitis, supraspinatus tendonitis, impingement syndrome and subacromial bursitis. Patients presenting with acute shoulder pain and a painful arc, who have limited pain control from analgesics/NSAIDs/Cox-2s, should be offered a steroid plus lidocaine injection into the subacromial bursa. This is to encourage exercise, so these patients should be given an exercise leaflet or additional physiotherapy. Most patients will not return for a further injection.

Glenohumeral capsulitis

Patients with a mixed picture of painful arc and glenohumeral capsulitis with limited pain control from prescribed medications should be given a choice of physiotherapy or steroid injection. Patients who have had this problem for less than 3 months tend to respond to steroid plus lidocaine injections, one into the subacromial bursa and one into the glenohumeral joint. It is essential to encourage exercise and use of the shoulder.

Around 10–15% of these patients will return for a second or third injection. These tend to be patients who have had shoulder pain for longer, have more disability and more yellow flags. They are also more frequent attenders for health care intervention.

The greater the degree of severity of the glenohumeral capsulitis, the less likelihood there is of the injections being effective. Such patients require more physiotherapy input but it is unclear whether it is the physiotherapy that is important or the psychological help that accompanies it (c.f., back pain management).

Acromioclavicular joint pain

Patients who point to the AC joint as the source of pain respond remarkably well to steroid plus lidocaine injection into this joint.

Wrist/thumb/hand problems
De Quervain's tenosynovitis

The classic features are:
- Redness of abductor pollicis longus and extensor pollicis brevis tendon sheaths,
- Swelling of these tendon sheaths, and
- Pain on use or tenderness on palpation over the tendons.

66 Tenosynovitis is a prescribed condition in the UK meaning that it is a compensatory occupational injury ... If this term is used, the patient should have the classic triad (redness, swelling, pain) 99

Tenosynovitis is a prescribed condition in the UK, meaning that it is a compensatory occupational injury, so beware of using the term De Quervain's tenosynovitis or tenosynovitis on a sick note. If this term is used, the patient should have the classic triad (redness, swelling, pain). Unless all three criteria are present, it is better to use the terms "thumb pain" or "peritendonitis crepitus", as crepitus is often felt on palpation or by the patient on use. Further confirmation of the diagnosis is by passive ulnar deviation of the wrist with the enclosed thumb.

Finkelstein's test

A positive test is produced when pain is elicited on the patient folding the thumb into the palm of the hand and encircling it with the fist, then passively deviating the wrist towards the ulnar side, i.e., away from the radial side. The differential diagnosis is OA of the thumb in the carpometacarpal (CMC) joint. Most patients under 45 years will

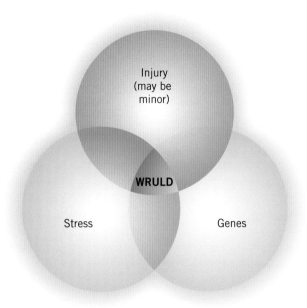

Fig. 21 The three components of work-related upper limb disorder (WRULD)

have thumb pain/peritendonitis crepitus and consideration of an overuse injury or work-related upper limb disorder (WRULD) is more appropriate than OA.

Work-related upper limb disorders

Many conditions that may be related to overuse also frequently occur in the general population, e.g., carpal tunnel syndrome, epicondylitis and some shoulder problems. If symptoms occur over a wide area, the term "non-specific work-related upper limb disorder" tends to be used. The term RSI (repetitive strain injury) is less likely to be used, but in the sports field, "overuse injury" may be used. Fig. 21 shows the components of WRULD.

- Musculoskeletal problems can be aggravated by work or exercise.
- If physical working conditions change, work may cause the musculoskeletal problem.
- Stress in the workplace or at home is another factor. It can be caused by stress factors such as an unsympathetic superior within the workplace, bullying and sex discrimination problems.
- There appears to be a genetic predisposition to WRULD, although there is little evidence to suggest that certain personality types are likely to suffer from it (see Reflex sympathetic dystrophy [RSD], page 54). Which came first, WRULD or the personality?
- Remember that pain is the major problem: there is not necessarily any serious damage to any specific tendon or structure. This means that the pain is out of all proportion to any damage.

❝ Most patients under 45 years will have thumb pain/ peritendonitis crepitus and consideration of an overuse injury or WRULD is more appropriate than OA ❞

- One way of explaining WRULD to patients is to suggest that their stress does not allow muscles to relax. They are continually tense, even during the night, which means that they have not "refuelled" overnight before the next day's work. No wonder patients experience pain.
- People at special risk are those in jobs with high rates of repetition or work involving abnormal lifting and using tools in unnatural positions, i.e., above shoulder height.
- Athletes are not immune, especially long-distance runners, nor are musicians, who perform at the speed dictated by the composer/conductor. String players develop shoulder problems and keyboard players develop hand problems. Dancers and athletes may develop compartment syndromes.

Common symptoms include:

- pain,
- cramp,
- muscle weakness,
- dropping objects, e.g., cups,
- pins and needles/paraesthesia,
- clumsiness,
- burning/unpleasant sensations (hyperalgesia).

These usually occur after performing a task or action for a certain length of time. Ask about what has changed, what new activity has been undertaken by the patient.

66 Common symptoms usually occur after performing a task or action for a certain length of time. Ask about what has changed, what new activity has been undertaken by the patient 99

Practical management

- Advise the patient to avoid the activity or change the movements around the activity.
- If symptoms start after 15 minutes, then advise a change of task at 10–12 minutes, returning after a 3–5-minute break. If the problem is back strain after 3 hours sitting down, advise a 5-minute break after $2\frac{1}{2}$ hours.
- Look at how stresses can be relieved or camouflaged. Advise no over-time work, and more weekend breaks or shorter holidays more regularly.
- Involve the company nurse, occupational therapist or doctor, where available; otherwise, obtain advice from or refer to the community physiotherapist and even the disability employment advisor.
- Advise about general health and fitness.
- Consider advising about the use of firm bandages or supports, which often give enough confidence to allow the patient to continue to work (see tennis elbow, page 56).
- Do not forget the comfort of a warm bowl of water for the hands or a hot bath once work is finished. Sometimes a cold pack works better than a hot pack.

- Appropriate local steroid injections may buy time or even alleviate the problem if performed in the early stages.
- Always use paracetamol as the drug of first choice, or paracetamol plus codeine or co-codamol, before considering prescribing NSAIDs, where appropriate.
- Recovery tends to be a function of how long the patient has had the problems. In general, recovery time = time condition has been present. The average time for a severe case of WRULD is 3–4 years.

Legal aspects of management

- Employers need to provide a well-designed working environment (Fig. 22).
- Employees are often interested in pursuing legal claims, although there is rarely a case. Employers usually follow the Health & Safety directives and are careful to check risk assessments in the work place and ensure that employees take regular breaks and/or changes of activity.

The onus is on the employee to prove:

- existence of a medical condition, as defined by the law, e.g., De Quervain's tenosynovitis,
- that the medical condition was caused by work activities,
- that the employer was negligent.

Problems in proving the above include:

- the employee's medical records must confirm that similar injuries have not happened previously,
- that the employee's hobbies or home activities have not contributed.

Carpal tunnel syndrome

The most common entrapment neuropathy is caused by increased pressure in the carpal tunnel. The pressure produces ischaemia of the median nerve, resulting in impaired nerve conduction that produces the symptoms of paraesthesia and pain. Initially, symptoms are intermittent and

> *Always use paracetamol as the drug of first choice, or paracetamol plus codeine or co-codamol, before considering prescribing NSAIDs, where appropriate*

> *Carpal tunnel pressure produces ischaemia of the median nerve, resulting in impaired nerve conduction that produces the symptoms of paraesthesia and pain*

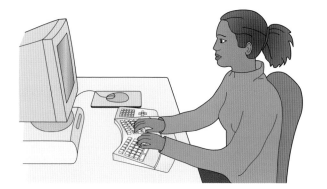

Fig. 22 Well-designed work desk. Reprinted from Work-Related Rheumatic Complaints, **arc** patient information leaflet.

the neurological findings are reversible. If there is prolonged elevation of pressure, there may be demyelination, the pins-and-needles symptom becomes constant and the muscle weakness becomes more severe. Conditions associated with carpal tunnel syndrome include:

- diabetes (6% of patients),
- hypothyroidism,
- WRULD,
- pregnancy,
- previous Colles' fracture,
- inflammatory arthritis.

Signs and symptoms

- More common in women, affecting all ages.
- Pain or aching and tingling and numbness.
- Usually worse in thumb and index and middle fingers (Fig. 23), but patients often do not differentiate the pins and needles into specific fingers and just report symptoms in the whole hand.
- Classically, symptoms are worse at night, interrupting sleep. Patients will hang the affected arm out of bed and shake it vigorously to relieve symptoms. This latter sign is said to be the most consistent and reliable and should always be asked about when taking a case history (sometimes called the "flick" sign).
- Symptoms may occur during the day, especially if it is WRULD. Up to 50% of patients will develop symptoms in the other hand.
- Late presentation shows signs of constant numbness, symptoms for more than 1 year, loss of sensibility at the finger ends and thenar muscular atrophy.

Tests for carpal tunnel syndrome include:

- Test for motor power for muscles innervated by the median nerve (Fig. 23). To test the Opponen's muscle, try to separate the tightly

66 Classically, symptoms are worse at night, interrupting sleep. Patients will hang the affected arm out of bed and shake it vigorously to relieve symptoms. This latter sign is said to be the most consistent and reliable and should always be asked about when taking a case history (sometimes called the "flick" sign) 99

Fig. 23 Carpal tunnel syndrome. Reprinted from Collected Reports on the Rheumatic Diseases, **arc.**

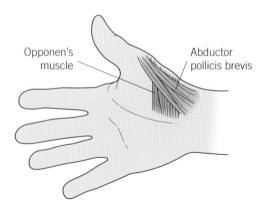

Opponen's muscle

Abductor pollicis brevis

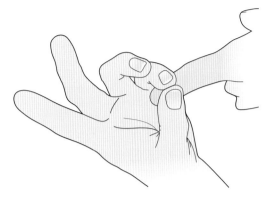

Fig. 24 Test for motor power in hand muscles: Opponen's muscle.
Reprinted from Collected Reports on the Rheumatic Diseases, **arc.**

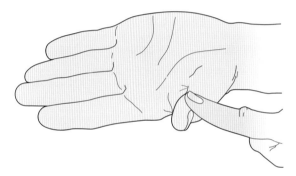

Fig. 25 Test for motor power in hand muscles: abductor pollicis brevis.
Reprinted from Collected Reports on the Rheumatic Diseases, **arc.**

opposed tips of the thumb and little fingers (Fig. 24). To test the abductor pollicis brevis, the patient places the back of the hand flat on a table and raises the thumb vertically while the movement is resisted by the examiner (Fig. 25).

- Phalen's sign: flexion of the wrist for 60 seconds produces pain or paraesthesia in the median nerve distribution.
- Tinel's sign: radiating paraesthesia in the fingers when tapped lightly with a tendon hammer over the median nerve at the wrist.

These tests tend to be positive when the condition is more severe and the diagnosis is more easily made. The "flick test" is more helpful for less severe cases, but the history gives the main clues and usually the diagnosis.

Practical management toolbox
Modification of activities
This should apply to all patients where possible. It is particularly important for any patient with elements of WRULD. Advice from a community or employment occupational therapist should be sought.

Splints (Futuro wrist splints)

These are excellent for alleviating symptoms in 80% of patients and are certainly the preferred treatment in patients who do not have abnormal signs but do have a positive history. Patients who are very apprehensive about injections or surgery may wish to try splints. It is important that splints are worn in the *neutral* position, not in extension. They can be obtained from physiotherapy/occupational therapy departments or ordered from the Mobilis catalogue.

Local corticosteroid injections

Of patients with symptoms and some signs, 75% respond to injections of corticosteroid into the carpal tunnel. Symptoms recur in more severe cases within 1 year. It is possible to give a repeat injection when symptoms recur or it may be advisable to consider surgical decompression. There are no randomized controlled trials (RCTs) assessing long-term outcomes of repeated injections compared to surgical decompression.

Surgical decompression

"Surgical release should be seriously considered where there are severe signs and symptoms suggesting axonal loss"

Surgical release should be driven by patient preference. It should be seriously considered where there are severe signs and symptoms suggesting axonal loss:

- constant numbness,
- symptoms > 1 year,
- loss of sensibility,
- thenar muscle atrophy.

There are different surgical techniques:

- traditional open procedure,
- endoscopic release, using one or two portals, which carries a higher risk of median nerve damage,
- mini-open release of the transverse carpal ligament.

NSAIDs/Cox-2s and other therapies

RCTs have shown no benefit with NSAIDs or diuretics over placebo. In the short term (2 weeks), oral steroids are better than placebo. In a small RCT, the same result was produced after 8 weeks. There are no long-term studies. Local steroid injections are better than oral prednisolone at 8–12 weeks. There are no studies on the use of intramuscular steroids.

Nerve conduction studies

This should not be routine and should only be undertaken where the diagnosis is uncertain and particularly when surgery is being contemplated.

Screening

Screening for diabetes and hypothyroidism should be undertaken.

Trigger finger/thumb

Trigger finger typically affects people over 30 years old and commonly affects the second finger. It may be related to a specific task when the flexor tendon has been minimally damaged and thickened, causing it to catch on the sheath. This nodule is often palpable. Classically, the finger is stuck down on waking in the morning and has to be forcibly straightened, causing pain and, often, an audible click.

Trigger thumb is a sesamoiditis, usually of the sesamoid bone. Palpation over this point is very painful. It is also probably related to overuse, especially gripping.

Practical management

Rarely will the alteration of activities solve these two conditions, nor do patients accept splints. Both respond very well to local corticosteroid.

"Rarely will the alteration of activities solve trigger finger/thumb"

Thumb injection

A 25-gauge (orange) needle is placed into or around the painful sesamoid. Occasionally, this needs to be repeated, presumably because either the injection was not accurate enough or because it failed to relieve the inflammation.

Finger injection

This is given into the tendon sheath and rarely needs to be repeated. Triggering usually stops in 3–4 days, certainly within 10 days. Orthopaedic surgeons advocate a percutaneous procedure that involves slipping a large 19-gauge needle down the tendon and rotating it at the level of the nodule. It does not appear to cause problems but until evidence is accrued, a 25-gauge needle should be the initial preferred option.

Dupuytren's contracture affecting the palmar fascia

- More common in men, with a genetic component.
- More commonly affects the ulnar side, often bilaterally.
- May affect the feet, and has an association with Peyronie's disease.
- Nodular thickening of the palmar fascia, drawing one or more fingers into flexion contracture.
- Runs a variable course and does not always require corrective surgery (see below).

Practical management
- Advice to stretch the fingers is always given and may help.
- The tendons themselves are not involved; there is a contracture of the connective tissues.
- In early Peyronie's disease, steroid injections are used. Early use of steroid injections into the contracting tissue may be tried for Dupuytren's contracture, but should be done before there is obvious flexion of the fingers. Use 0.2mL lidocaine plus 0.3mL steroid with a 25-guage needle inserted into either the contracting tissue or the tendon sheath above the contractures.
- Progression of the contractures is variable but patients should be referred for surgery before there is marked flexion contracture, otherwise plastic surgery will be required for the accompanying skin defect.
- To obtain best results, the affected finger and flexor tendon *must* be stretched from the third day after surgery. The patient must be encouraged to do this for themselves and not to rely on an early appointment with a physiotherapist. Remember, the tendon is not involved in the process.

❝ To obtain best results, the affected finger and flexor tendon must be stretched from the third day after surgery. The patient must be encouraged to do this for themselves and not to rely on an early appointment with a physiotherapist. Remember, the tendon is not involved in the process ❞

Reflex sympathetic dystrophy

RSD is a descriptive term applied to a symptom complex characterized by severe pain, swelling and autonomic vasomotor dysfunction (sweating and abnormal blood flow). It is not necessary for all components to be present.

The full clinical picture is uncommon but minor degrees, where not all components are present, are often seen in primary care. It is usually seen after trauma or immobilization of a limb. The patient does not want to use the joint or limb and so appears to want to prolong the "injury". This "insult" may be minor: it can be compared with injuries in childhood where a child needs encouragement to use a leg again, even after a minor bump. In RSD, this "worry about harm" seems to have become pathological. There is an element of RSD in WRULD and the two conditions may overlap.

Minor degrees of RSD are seen in children. Prospective studies have found incidences of more than 30% following Colles' or tibial fractures.

Precipitating factors
There are three broad groups:
- trauma, including fractures and events such as arthroscopy,
- central nervous system or spinal disorders, even following lumbar spine surgery,
- visceral lesions, for example following myocardial infarction.

In some cases, it is difficult to identify an underlying cause, especially in children.

Is there a personality trait?

It is difficult to know which comes first, the RSD or the marked behavioural change. As yet, there is no definite evidence that certain personality traits predispose to the development of RSD. Neurogenic pain may induce illness behaviour so that doctors may tend to disbelieve patients, increasing their distress.

Clinical features

RSD generally affects the extremities, i.e., hand, foot, ankle and knee. There is also a variant called shoulder hand syndrome.

- pain, usually distally, described as burning,
- tenderness, often hyperaesthesia and allodynia,
- oedema,
- vasomotor and sudomotor changes,
- weakness, tremor, muscle spasm,
- dystrophic changes of nails and skin,
- contractures.

Have a high index of suspicion for RSD, especially if the patient has pain distally, spreading proximally and the pain is burning in character (different from the pain of injury). Be aware of allodynia (a stimulus that does not usually produce pain) and hyperpathia (exaggerated reaction to a painful stimulus). The tenderness may be generalized and there is often oedema. Try not to miss the vasomotor changes; the area is initially often warm, red or mottled or cyanotic with increased sweating. Later, the limb can be cold, dry and pale. These changes happen in the first 3–6 months. Hopefully, recovery or referral will have occurred before the later stages of muscle tremor, weakness and spasm. The irreversible changes of atrophy and contracture, even ankylosis of the joint, are rarely seen in primary care.

Differential diagnosis and investigations

These red flags need to be excluded:

- more trauma,
- non-accidental injury in children,
- cellulitis,
- inflammatory arthritis,
- malignancy.

Usually, a careful history will give the diagnosis. The only worthwhile, easily available investigation is a dual-energy X-ray absorptiometry (DEXA) scan, which should only be required for patients who are not responding to early treatment and require secondary referral. DEXA scanning is usually organized within secondary care and generally shows osteoporosis of the affected area.

"RSD generally affects the extremities, i.e., hand, foot, ankle and knee"

55

Practical management
- Early clinical suspicion and diagnosis is the key, as treatment is usually unsuccessful in the late stages of RSD.
- Physiotherapy, intensive mobilisation.
- Pain relief to aid mobilization is important and if there is osteoporosis, bisphosphonates are useful. Some doctors use these drugs early for pain relief, to prevent osteoporosis and to aid physiotherapy.
- Other measures such as sympathetic blocks are for secondary care.

Elbow problems
Tennis/golfers elbow (lateral/medial epicondylitis)
This affects 1–3% of adults per year and accounts for 4–7 patients per 1000 GP appointments. Typically, tennis or golfers elbow lasts 6–24 months.

Symptoms and signs
- Pain over lateral/medial epicondyle made worse by pressure.
- Pain over the lateral humeral epicondyle on resisted palmar flexion of the wrist = golfers elbow (Fig. 26a).
- Pain over the medial humeral epicondyle on resisted dorsiflexion of the wrist = tennis elbow (Fig. 26b).

Fig. 26 Tests for golfer's and tennis elbow.
Reprinted from Standards in Rheumatology: A Suggested Management Plan for Some Common Conditions in Rheumatology, The Medicine Group 1987.

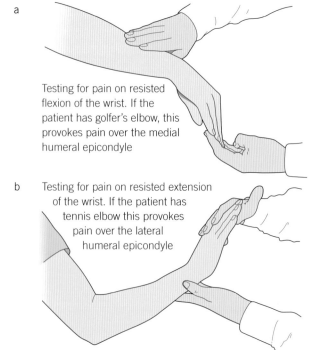

a

Testing for pain on resisted flexion of the wrist. If the patient has golfer's elbow, this provokes pain over the medial humeral epicondyle

b Testing for pain on resisted extension of the wrist. If the patient has tennis elbow this provokes pain over the lateral humeral epicondyle

Percentage of patients successfully treated after 52 weeks
Injections 69% (n = 43) Physiotherapy 91% (n = 58) Wait and see 83% (n = 49)

Fig. 27 Percentage of patients successfully treated after 52 weeks. Data modified from Smidt N, et al. Lancet 2002;359:657–62.

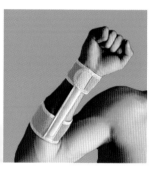

Fig. 28 Vulkan Medisplint double-strap elbow support. Reprinted from the Mobilis catalogue.

Treatment

Fig. 27 shows the percentage of patients who responded successfully to the various treatments after 52 weeks.

- Corticosteroid and lidocaine injection, given into the tenderest point, preferably down to the periosteum. A fan distribution gives good results. Injections work well for patients who have had the complaint for less than 6 weeks. Injections also give good short-term results for more chronic symptoms but poorer long-term relief.
- Physiotherapy: patients who have experienced lateral elbow pain for more than 6 weeks do best over the longer term with physiotherapy treatment or a wait and see policy. There is no statistical difference between these two options.
- If a patient presents with an acute episode of elbow pain, an injection is probably indicated. Otherwise, the patient requires encouragement to use the elbow. This may be achieved by physiotherapy or supplying a tennis elbow support. The easiest to wear is the Vulkan double-strap support type, available in four sizes (Fig. 28). These cannot be inadvertently worn over the tenderest point. Unfortunately, the simple variety with one strap, often supplied by physiotherapists, is frequently repositioned by the patient and placed over the maximum point of tenderness. This is incorrect and probably the reason for its high non-effective rate. The elbow support merely allows the patient to use the elbow normally again

❝ Patients who have experienced lateral elbow pain for more than 6 weeks do best over the longer term with physiotherapy treatment or a wait and see policy ❞

and probably nothing more. The essential point is that the elbow support should not be too large, otherwise it will restrict elbow or wrist movement. The patient should use the support for 24 hours, i.e., day and night, for 3 weeks and then most of the time for the following 3 months (some patients wear it only at night).

Olecranon bursitis

This is a common inflammatory bursitis, usually caused by trauma (commonly called boozer's elbow). It may result from an arthropathy, e.g., RA or gout. It is rarely septic. There is localized swelling and tenderness over the olecranon bursa.

Treatment

Remove the fluid by aspiration. Enter laterally from an area of skin not involved with the inflamed bursa so that this tract acts as a valve and the needle tract is less likely to become a discharging sinus.

Ankle and foot problems
Biomechanics

The foot and ankle with all their joints, tendons and muscles are a superb biomechanical structure.

- There is some movement in every direction.
- This has the potential to cause problems with the stability required for weight bearing and propulsion.
- All except the phalangeal joints have one major movement and movement in other planes.
- Only the phalangeal joints are restricted to movement in one plane. This is required for greater precision of movement.
- This system has two advantages:
  - Forces can be dissipated throughout the system of joints, tendons, capsules and muscles, so limiting joint and tissue injury.
  - If injury (or a congenital or surgical problem) occurs, the system allows some compensatory movement at other joints.
- The ankle and foot may need to compensate for problems of the back, hip or knee.

Foot arches

Flying buttresses and arched bridges are an effective and economical way of transferring loads and stresses. The longitudinal foot arch is basically a flying buttress and the transverse arch is an arch or suspension bridge (Fig. 29). These arches need looking after and all biomechanical assessments and treatments are in some way related to this.

> *Flying buttresses and arched bridges are an effective and economical way of transferring loads and stresses. The longitudinal foot arch is basically a flying buttress and the transverse arch is an arch or suspension bridge*

a Longitudinal arch

b Transverse arch

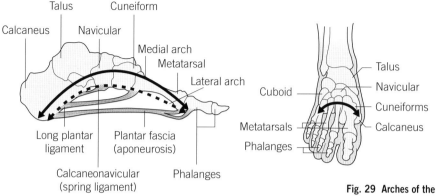

Fig. 29 Arches of the foot. Reprinted from the University of Bath Diploma, Module 5 – Lower Limb.

Longitudinal arch

This has three major supporting ligaments giving it elasticity and flexibility (Fig. 29a). If it collapses, the biomechanical consequences are:

- a flat foot,
- pronation,
- eversion of the heel,
- tarsal bone problems; callosities may form over the tarsal heads.

Transverse arch

This arch relates to the forefoot (Fig. 29b). The metatarsals are arranged along it, so that the arch takes the load. If the arch is lost, there is less room for the metatarsal heads in the shoe and the forefoot spreads and the foot becomes broader. Lack of room in the shoe causes the metatarsal heads to rub together, squeezing the digital nerve and causing metatarsalgia or a neuroma. Other associated problems will be the production of hammer toes (change in pulleys and anatomical relationships). Loss of the transverse arch may be secondary to loss of the longitudinal arch and in this situation it often leads to, or exacerbates, the development of hallux valgus.

Types of feet

- high arched feet (pes cavus or supinated foot) (Fig. 30a),
- flat (pronated feet) (Fig. 30c).

There are three types of flat (pronated) foot:

- Dynamic flat foot: Many individuals have flat feet. This may be of no consequence in children or in people with hypermobility so long as the arch reconstitutes itself fully when the patient stands on

a Supination   b Normal footprint   c Pronation

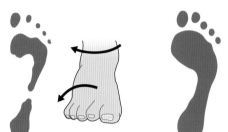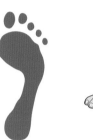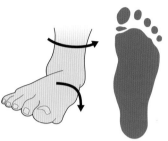

Fig. 30 Types of feet.
Reprinted from the
University of Bath
Diploma, Module 5 –
Lower Limb.

tiptoe. This is a dynamic flat foot. No treatment is necessary unless there are symptoms, which usually occur in older patients with hypermobility as the muscles become weaker. A sorbothane arch support (obtained from Mobilis) will ease most symptoms.

- Static flat foot: If ligaments become strained, causing pain, or if there is pain from muscle fatigue, then the aches and pains may make standing intolerable for the patient. These problems are more common in hypermobile patients and, if they progress and become chronic, there may well be chronic spasm. On examination, there is pain on inversion of the foot and tenderness on palpation of the tendons. This is described as a static flat foot because it is still possible to relax and move the foot.
- Rigid foot: The foot can no longer be relaxed and deformities are permanent. The classic example is the rheumatoid foot.

The consequences of a high arched foot are:
- some degree of hammer or claw toes,
- heel displaced medially (inversion),
- less flexibility and less articular movement than the normal foot,
- tendency to calluses over metatarsal heads and toes (these may cause major problems for runners and walkers),
- symptoms of discomfort and aching.

The severest forms are usually congenital and occur in association with neurological disorders such as spina bifida and Friedrich's ataxia.

Examination
Hindfoot movements
The ankle joint is a hinge between the tibia and fibula and the trochlea of the talus, allowing only flexion of 55° and extension (also called dorsiflexion) of 15°. To examine, grip the lower leg above the malleoli from behind and move the midfoot and forefoot with the other hand to assess flexion and extension (Fig. 31).

a Plantar flexion

b Dorsiflexion (extension)

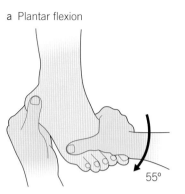

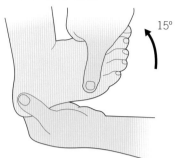

15°

55°

Fig. 31 Hindfoot plantar flexion and dorsiflexion. Reprinted from the University of Bath Diploma, Module 5 – Lower Limb.

a

b

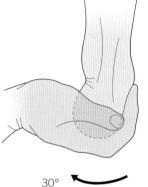

30°

20°

Subtalar joint movement

Also called the talocalcaneal joint, this lies between the concave facet of the talus and the upper posterior surface of the calcaneus. It allows inversion (supination) and eversion (pronation). To examine, grip the lower leg to stabilize it and use the other hand to rock the calcaneus from side to side (Fig. 32). Inversion is normally 30° and eversion is 20°.

Fig. 32 Subtalar joint inversion and eversion. Reprinted from the University of Bath Diploma, Module 5 – Lower Limb.

Midfoot tarsal joints (metatarsus)

These are a composite set of joints allowing inversion and eversion at the midfoot. There is more than one axis of movement, giving rise to problems in the forefoot or hindfoot.

Metatarsal squeeze

Gently grasp across the metatarsal/midfoot and if this causes pain there is probably inflammation in one or more MTP joints. Use a finger and thumb to identify which joints are causing the pain and to

61

detect signs of inflammation in individual joints of the forefoot. To examine for movement, stabilize the lower leg and calcaneus with one hand (immobilize the hindfoot) and with the other hand, rotate the midfoot into inversion (30°) and eversion (40°).

First metatarsophalangeal joint (forefoot movement)

To examine, stabilize the midfoot and forefoot with one hand and use the other hand to move the big toe into extension (80°) and flexion (35°).

Achilles tendon problems

Signs and symptoms

- pain, swelling and tenderness of the tendon above the insertion into the calcaneus,
- commonly seen in relation to sports activities.

Practical management

- Pain relief (analgesics or NSAIDs) plus self-administered Achilles tendon stretching exercises (see **arc** website, Hands On, Plantar Fasciitis) usually suffices. Local heat and ultrasound are useful additional treatments.
- Advice to stretch the tendon before exercise. Consider the use of ice packs following exercise, with or without NSAIDs.
- Check trainers, shoes and walking boots for precipitating factors such as protruding stitching, folds in material or Achilles protectors.

Chronic Achilles tendonitis/paratendonitis (see Fig. 59 page 120 and page 119)

❝ Chronic Achilles tendonitis/ paratendonitis is classically seen in postmenopausal, overweight women who wear only slip-on shoes ❞

- Classically seen in postmenopausal, overweight women who wear only slip-on shoes. It is a biomechanical problem due to forward movement of the centre of gravity. Patients have static flat feet and an excess strain is placed on the Achilles tendon, especially the lateral side.
- Practical treatment is $3/4$ sorbothane insoles (see page 119) and stretching exercises (appendix 5 page 184). Steroid injection gives only short-term relief. Advice about losing weight is rarely adhered to. In a few patients with extremely chronic tendonitis/paratendonitis, surgical help may be required.

Achilles rupture

Rupture tends to happen when muscles are fatigued, especially in sports people or the elderly, or as a side effect of the antibiotic ciprofloxacin.

Clinical presentation

- sudden pain, as if kicked in the back of the lower leg,

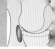

- difficult to stand on tiptoe,
- defect may be palpable.

For the squeeze test, the patient should be relaxed and lying in the prone position with the feet over the end of a couch. When the calves are squeezed, the normal foot will plantar flex while the injured one will not.

Practical management

- Orthopaedic referral and probably surgery may be necessary for the young sports person. Conservative strapping is the treatment for elderly, less active patients.
- Early physiotherapy is required to help stretch the healing, contracting tendon. Early stretching should prevent a recurrence of the rupture.

Plantar fasciitis

- More commonly seen in middle-aged to elderly patients who are overweight and have developed a pronated foot.
- Pain and tenderness are present at the anteromedial aspect of the calcaneus where the plantar fascia is inserted.
- In sports people, this is often seen with a high instep and may be a more chronic, long-term problem.

Practical management

- Treatment includes stretching, massage, ultrasound and the help of a sports physiotherapist.
- The biomechanical treatment includes wearing a sorbothane arch support with a heel pad (Fig. 58 page 118) and stretching the plantar fascia and Achilles tendon (see appendix 5).
- Local steroid injections are rarely indicated.
- Be aware that an enthesopathy may present with Achilles tendonitis, heel pain or plantar fasciitis.
- Bruised heel syndrome (heel pad pain) is more posterior on the calcaneus. Biomechanical treatment is to wear shock-absorbing heels and shoes.

Tarsal tunnel syndrome

- Often overlooked in primary care.
- Symptoms are poorly localized heel or foot pain.
- There may be a burning sensation, especially in the toes, and this may spread into the calf.
- Caused by pressure on the posterior tibial nerve by the flexor retinaculum (attached to the medial malleolus and the calcaneus) (Fig. 33).

> ❝ *Plantar fasciitis is more commonly seen in middle-aged to elderly patients who are overweight and have developed a pronated foot* ❞

Fig. 33 Tarsal tunnel.
Reprinted from the
University of Bath
Diploma, Module 5 –
Lower Limb.

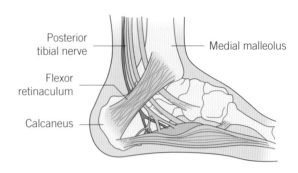

Posterior
tibial nerve — Medial malleolus

Flexor
retinaculum

Calcaneus

- Percussion along the nerve route (Tinel's sign) elicits the pain.
- Treatment is a steroid injection below and behind the medial malleolus. Biomechanical assessment is also indicated to correct any pronation, valgus, etc.

Metatarsalgia

- This is pain and tenderness (sensation of walking on pebbles) over the metatarsal head region of the foot. The metatarsal heads should be arranged along the transverse arch but due to muscle weakness the arch may flatten. This weakness may be seen in hypermobile female patients who have gone through the menopause.
- RA may present with foot pain, especially metatarsalgia.

❝The metatarsal heads should be arranged along the transverse arch but due to muscle weakness the arch may flatten ❞

Morton's neuroma

This is a degenerative rather than proliferative process. The common digital nerve to the 3rd/4th interspace is most often involved.

- Common in women.
- Burning pain in the metatarsal heads radiating into the toe(s). May radiate proximally.
- Pain made worse by walking and tight-fitting shoes.
- Relief obtained if the shoes are removed and the foot is massaged.

Practical management

This should be biomechanical. Surgery should be the last resort as it will relieve the pain but will leave the toes numb.

- Change to wider fitting shoes.
- Insoles, to correct any pronation and metatarsalgia, may relieve the problems.
- Steroid injections should be tried next.

Hallux valgus

A common deformity caused by swelling on the medial aspect of the first metatarsal head and a broadening forefoot, usually caused by loss of the transverse arch. The hallux dislocates and moves into valgus; a bunion invariably occurs. In some patients, the biomechanical forces change so that the weight goes through the second toe, producing a callosity and a hammer toe. These forces displace the first toe so that it over- or under-rides the second toe and, incredibly, this may all be asymptomatic.

Practical management

Treatment should be primarily biomechanical. Surgery should be a last resort when the pain continues despite adequate conservative treatment.
* wider, deeper shoes,
* insoles to correct the over-pronation,
* steroid injections may help.

Hallux rigidus

There is restricted movement, usually caused by OA at the first MTP joint. Dorsiflexion is reduced so that the patient complains of pain and stiffness on walking. If a callosity develops under the metatarsal head, obtaining comfortable shoes may be difficult.

Practical management

* Insoles promote plantar flexion and reduce pronation.
* Steroid injections can augment pain relief.
* Surgery for joint fusion is a last resort.

Sprained ankle

An inversion injury to the lateral component is the most common injury. Many of these will be seen and treated in primary care. Only the severest require referral to accident and emergency for X-ray.
* Common in all age groups.
* The usual stress is plantar flexion and inversion causing injury to one or more parts of the lateral ligament.
* The lateral ligament has three parts/bands (Fig. 34).
    - anterior talofibular,
    - calcaneofibular,
    - posterior talofibular.

The anterior talofibular and calcaneofibular bands are more commonly injured. Injuries require grading for practical management:
* Grade I: local tenderness only.
* Grade II: tenderness, swelling and restriction of movement; pain on weight bearing.

❝Only the severest require referral to accident and emergency for X-ray❞

65

Fig. 34 Lateral ligament complex of the ankle joint. Reprinted by permission of Oxford University Press from Hutson MA, Sports Injuries: Recognition and Management, OUP 1990.

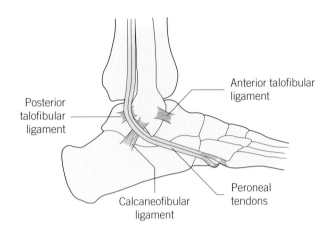

- Grade III: swelling, tenderness, severe pain, early bruising and difficulty or inability to bear weight.

Approach to management

Where possible, this should be self-management with expert support. Immediate measures are to:

- check that the joint is not unstable,
- X-ray only Grade III and refer to an orthopaedic surgeon.

In the first 24–48 hours:

- rest,
- elevation: raise the end of the bed (on bricks),
- ice, wrapped in a towel, placed on the joint for 10–20 minutes at a time: often excellent for pain control,
- compression, using a tubigrip (doubled), a crepe bandage or a neoprene ankle support,
- NSAIDs where appropriate (use Cox-2s if > 65 years), at least twice the maintenance dose for the first 2 days (this is a similar regime to that for an acute attack of gout).

On days 2–7:

- Continue NSAIDs/Cox-2s in maintenance doses.
- Patient to start modified weight bearing wearing ankle support.
- Use a modified range of motion exercises, especially lateral inversion. To do this, the patient stands in a doorway so that the body weight can be supported, then the ankle is moved to discomfort. This should be done from day 3, to stop contraction of the healing ligaments. In this way, greater strength and less shortening occurs, leading to less chance of recurrence.

> **❝** Ice, wrapped in a towel, placed on the joint for 10–20 minutes at a time: often excellent for pain control **❞**

On days 7–28:
- Progressive mobilization, strengthening and stretching exercises should be carried out.
- An ankle support should be worn for sports activities until the patient is fully fit.
- Remember that most injuries occur in the last quarter of play in competitive sports and near the end of a walk or the day's activities in the active elderly.

General tips on practical management
- Advice regarding shoes should always be given but may not be accepted, so compromises may be necessary. Commonly available sensible shoes include: Hotter, Ecco, Padders, Clarke's Springer Sandals or any make of trainers.
- Thin sorbothane insoles are a reasonable compromise that will usually fit in dress shoes and help to relieve discomfort and aches.
- Sorbothane arch supports are often invaluable for static flat feet. They are the ideal way to compensate for biomechanical foot problems of patients with plantar fasciitis. Importantly, they make steel-capped work boots much more comfortable (Fig. 58 page 118).
- Sorbothane $^3/_4$ arch supports are the compromise for patients who only wear slip-on shoes and will never change to ones that give more support, such as lace ups. These patients are usually overweight and often have difficulty fastening shoes (see Fig. 59 page 120). The $^3/_4$ arch supports do not prevent the toes being squashed into these shoes and therefore the patients will use them (see page 119).
- Physiotherapy, NSAIDs/Cox-2s and steroid injections may help. Ultrasound is unlikely to be beneficial.

> *Advice regarding shoes should always be given but may not be accepted, so compromises may be necessary*

Osteoarthritis
OA is the single biggest cause of joint pain and physical disability in primary care. Be cautious if:
- the patient is < 45 years: look for other causes,
- it is not the usual joints (hands, knees, hips): think again,
- the joint is swollen and hot: it may be gout or pseudogout,
- the patient has swollen osteoarthritic hands or a marked loss of function: could this be RA on a background of OA?
- there is generalized pain/pain all over: could this be fibromyalgia/chronic pain?

OA is a dynamic condition where there is breakdown and repair. Breakdown occurs in the cartilage and bone. In articular cartilage, it occurs in focal areas where there are changes in proteoglycan and water content and chondrocyte activity. The articular cartilage becomes

> *OA is the single biggest cause of joint pain and physical disability in primary care*

> *OA is a dynamic condition where there is breakdown and repair*

roughened and less able to withstand the forces applied to it, so wears away more easily. This process can extend into the bone, where the normal repair mechanism becomes overwhelmed and there is a change to remodelling and increased blood supply. The joint becomes wider (squarer) because of the osteophytes and the underlying bone has areas of sclerosis and bone cysts. It is possible that this process itself leads to further progression. Bone cysts, which appear in the bone below areas where there is no cartilage, lead to the characteristic changes seen on X-ray. Degradation products accumulate in the synovial fluid and may lead to an inflammatory response in the synovial lining, producing effusions. It is difficult to know whether the changes of OA start with changes in the synovial fluid or whether they are the consequence of the cartilage and bone changes. The synovial lining and fluid appear to have hormonal and messenger functions. Hyaluronan, the main constituent, has a high molecular weight giving it shock-absorbing, lubrication and possibly pain-relieving properties. In OA, the molecular weight of hyaluronan decreases.

❝ Not everyone develops OA, therefore it is not an inevitable event of ageing. Clinically, around 10% of patients will seek help for their arthritis but only 10% of these will require joint replacements ❞

Who develops clinical signs of osteoarthritis?

Not everyone develops OA, therefore it is not an inevitable event of ageing. Clinically, around 10% of patients will seek help for their arthritis but only 10% of these will require joint replacements. The knee joint probably causes the most disability in the community (Fig. 35).

Risk factors for development of knee and hip osteoarthritis

For the knee, these include:
- presence of Heberden's nodes,
- female gender,
- increasing age,
- obesity,
- internal derangement and instability,
- occupations involving repetitive knee bending,
- intensive sports activities, e.g., professional football.

Fig. 35 Prevalence of knee pain in an elderly population of 100,000 aged > 55 years.
Reprinted with permission from Elsevier: Elliot AM et al, *Lancet* 1999;354:1248–52.

Prevalence of knee pain in an elderly population of 100,000 aged > 55 years
25,000 will have knee pain for 4 weeks in any 1 year
4000 who consult a doctor with knee pain in any 1 year will be diagnosed with OA
1500 people with severely painful and disabling knee pain will be diagnosed with OA
OA = osteoarthritis

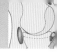

For the hip, these include:
- caucasian race,
- increasing age, although less than for knee OA. In some families, successive generations develop hip problems at an early age. Both genders can be affected,
- certain occupations, e.g., farming,
- sports, especially elite athletes,
- congenital and childhood hip disease, e.g., Legg-Perthes' disease, slipped femoral epiphysis, congenital dislocation of the hip and forms of dysplasia.

Clinical patterns in osteoarthritis
- Middle-aged to elderly woman typically have OA of hands and knees, clinically more severe in overweight patients.
- Younger men (often < 50 years) typically have OA of one joint, usually the hip.
- Middle-aged to older men typically have OA of one knee, invariably with a history of trauma.
- Elderly women typically have generalized OA of many joints, e.g., shoulders, hips, knees, hands and feet, often with cool effusions in the knees. The OA is progressive but all grades of severity are seen.

❝Younger men (often < 50 years) typically have OA of one joint, usually the hip ❞

The five clinical patterns of hand osteoarthritis
Examination of patients who have hand OA will differentiate five patterns (reprinted from Dickson J and Hosie G, Your Questions Answered – Osteoarthritis, Churchill Livingstone 2003):
- Heberden's/Bouchard's nodes,
- squaring of the first CMC thumb joint,
- thick stiff fingers,
- painful swollen knuckles or painful swollen knuckles and thumbs,
- deformed hands with good function.

Type I: Heberden's and Bouchard's nodes
- Patients may present with painful nodes, usually only when the nodes are developing. The nodes may be inflamed and swollen.
- Finger and thumb movements are not affected.
- Grip is not affected and function only minimally affected.
- In the very elderly, gout may superimpose on the distal interphalangeal nodes and joints.
- Treatment is rarely required. Topical NSAIDs may help or, rarely, a small quantity of triamcinolone can be injected.

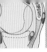

Type II: Squaring of the first carpometacarpal thumb joint

- thumb pain, which is use related,
- square CMC joint,
- dominant hand affected first,
- patient's grip and power grip affected so that twisting grip is painful,
- often no other joint affected,
- usually excellent response to steroid injections.

CMC splints may be used for hobbies, e.g., gardening.

Type III: Stiff, thick fingers

- wide and thicker fingers,
- distal interphalangeal (DIP), interphalangeal (IP) and metacarpophalangeal (MCP) joints may show squaring,
- thumb joints usually spared,
- function and movements, especially apposition of fingers into the palm of the hand, greatly affected by increased tissue in and around the flexor sheaths,
- usually both hands affected to a varying degree,
- holding golf clubs, tools and cups difficult,
- this is not the same as Dupuytren's contracture,

If seen early enough, i.e., before they have given up golf, injections into the flexor sheaths may restore function and grip.

Type IV(a): Painful swollen knuckles

- painful MCP joints, usually of the index and middle fingers,
- moderate inflammatory swelling of the involved MCP joints,
- joints painful to palpation as well as movement,
- thumb CMC joints often painful but rarely inflamed,
- grip severely affected so patient has great difficulty with cups, cutlery and buttons,
- commonly seen in people who knit.

❝ MCP joints respond well to steroid injections, which may be given intermittently ❞

MCP joints respond well to steroid injections, which may be given intermittently.

Type IV(b): Painful swollen knuckles and thumbs

- more severe presentation of Type IV(a),
- most MCP and first CMC joints painful and swollen,
- IP joints also painful and swollen,
- both hands generally equally affected and swollen,
- gripping and power grip difficult and extremely painful,
- no constitutional upset (in contrast to RA),

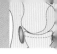

- no sweaty palms (in contrast to RA),
- both men and women affected; usually seen in people who work manually.

There are too many joints to inject. Most patients respond well to small doses of sulphasalazine (1g), though a few require 3g daily. Hydroxychloroquine is an alternative (200mg, 5 days/week).

Type V: Deformed hands with good function

- hands show ulnar deviation of joints and ulnar drift,
- all joints are affected,
- usually have both Heberden's and Bouchard's nodes,
- swollen MCP joints and square first CMC joints,
- wrist joints may be involved showing limited, painful movement; there may even be some ankylosis of the wrist joints,
- can be mistaken for RA but there is little loss of function (c.f., RA), grip strength is retained, flares are caused by knocks of working; flares respond to analgesics or an appropriate steroid injection and all inflammatory markers are negative.

X-ray reports may point to erosion in unstable DIP, but these are central (c.f., peripheral in RA), so view X-rays or ask for clarification to avoid erroneous diagnosis or treatment.

Obviously, not all patients fit into these categories: OA does not have a single cause. Genetics play a significant role: siblings of patients undergoing hip or knee replacements have a higher risk of developing OA (knee, x 3; hip, x 5). The role of trauma, especially in genetically susceptible individuals, must not be underestimated and probably accounts for a great number of patients presenting in primary care with a plethora of single-joint OA.

Necessary orthopaedic operations on the knee may lead to accelerated OA of the incident knee but also have an effect on the non-operated knee. This is trauma and genetic factors working together.

Metabolic insults are likely to play a part. Diabetic patients tend to develop shoulder problems, usually capsulitis, and many develop stiff joints as the diabetes progresses. However, there are no data to compare the incidence of OA in diabetics against the general population. Alcoholics appear to have an increased incidence of large-joint problems. Hypermobility is grossly under-reported. It affects peripheral joints, one side of the body or just one joint and is rarely recorded by doctors, though patients with joint pain may be labelled as having OA. Some patients with subluxed CMC joints who require joint fusion probably have an element of hypermobility.

> *Necessary orthopaedic operations on the knee may lead to accelerated OA of the incident knee but also have an effect on the non-operated knee. This is trauma and genetic factors working together*

71

What factors modify the development of osteoarthritis?

The genetics cannot be modified but susceptible families may consider certain options. Members of farming families with early hip replacements may wish to consider other occupations. Obesity is a factor that can be modified but most patients find it almost impossible to lose weight. OA occurs more commonly in the overweight and excess weight precedes the development of knee OA. Obesity also has an association with hip OA but this is not as strong as with knee OA. Vitamins C and D may affect the occurrence and progression of OA.

❝Pattern recognition is most important in helping recognise OA. If the pattern is not a good match, consider an alternative diagnosis ❞

Clinical pattern of osteoarthritis

Pattern recognition is most important in helping recognise OA. If the pattern is not a good match, consider an alternative diagnosis. No diagnostic or laboratory tests or X-rays conclusively confirm or exclude OA, although tests may help confirm an alternative diagnosis.

- usually > 50 years,
- use-related knee pain on walking or standing,
- morning stiffness rarely lasts longer than 30 minutes, compared to 45 minutes or longer in RA,
- joint stiffening after prolonged inactivity,
- crepitus when joint is moved,
- joint becomes harder and more square due to osteophytes,
- joint movement may change, i.e., loss of flexion or extension,
- effusion is cool and rarely large,
- sometimes the joint is tender on palpation, especially the joint line,

Fig. 36 Common painful conditions of the knee at different ages

Age	Articular	Periarticular	Referred
Children	Osteochondritis dissecans (M > F) Meniscal lesions Juvenile chronic arthritis Anterior knee pain syndrome (F > M) (hypermobility)	Bursitis Osgood-Schlatter	Hip disease
Young adults	Meniscal injury Cruciate ligament injury Inflammatory arthritis (reactive M > F, rheumatoid arthritis F > M) Anterior knee pain syndrome F > M) (hypermobility)	Fractures Collateral ligament injuries Bursitis	Hip disease
Adults > 45	Osteoarthritis (F > M) Fractures Meniscal injury	Bursitis	Hip disease

- often pain on palpitation over the anserine bursa or insertion of the medial collateral ligament,
- pain over the trochanteric bursa in hip OA,
- joint deformity occurs occasionally, classically varus deformity (bow legs),
- loss of muscles around the joint, e.g., poor quadriceps, is probably the cause of the feeling of insecurity (knee feeling as if it will give way).

Joint pain:
- may start insidiously as a vague ache after use or may accompany a viral infection,
- becomes more persistent in and around the joint,
- becomes an intermittent acute stabbing pain,
- becomes constant (night and day) in severe OA.

❝Joint pain may start insidiously as a vague ache after use or may accompany a viral infection ❞

Differential diagnosis

This includes common painful conditions of the knee at different ages (Fig. 36). Consider an alternative diagnosis when the following applies:
- patient < 45 years, especially females,
- patient ill or febrile (sepsis, gout or viral arthralgia),
- major loss of function plus inflammation of joints (RA),
- less commonly affected joints involved, e.g., wrist, ankle, elbow and shoulder,
- pain all over and tender points elicited (fibromyalgia/chronic pain),
- poorly controlled gout, with more chronic rather than acute attacks; patient on allopurinol (perhaps thiazide or low-dose aspirin has been prescribed recently),
- psychosocial problems in a patient with previously well-controlled, mild/moderate OA; emotion affects pain,
- patient > 70 years (pseudogout could cause severe pain),
- diffuse muscle pains over the shoulders and pelvic girdles (PMR); check ESR and consider a trial of steroids (15mg).

Investigations are required to exclude differential diagnosis, when necessary. X-rays should not be routine as they equate with clinical signs only in severe OA. See pages 17–22 for further discussion of investigations.

Management

This is discussed in more detail elsewhere in this book. Always consider:
- education and reassurance (page 114),
- general management – lifestyle, shoes, etc. (page 119),
- non-pharmalogical management (page 119),
- pharmalogical treatment (page 124),
- surgery (page 138).

Chronic pain

Chronic pain is common and a major challenge to the primary care team. It should be considered as a distinct entity even when associated with many of the common conditions seen in primary care. Chronic pain may be an entity in itself and can, if recognised soon enough, be treated effectively.

It is important that patients with chronic pain are diagnosed as soon as possible so that management can be implemented. This will hopefully prevent the common scenarios often associated with these patients.

Scenarios of chronic pain

- Patients with chronic pain use primary care services up to five times more often than the general population.
- They are over-prescribed.
- They are over-investigated.
- They are over-referred.
- They use up vast amounts of health care resources.

This sequence of events can lead to frustration on both the patient's and the doctor's part and to difficult relationships between the patient and medical advisors. Health staff may consider that the patient is looking for other gain, for example social security benefits, and sometimes feel that the symptoms are not genuine.

Pain definition

Pain is very subjective and any definition needs to acknowledge its multifactorial nature. The definition of the International Association for the Study of Pain is most widely accepted: "pain is an unpleasant sensory and emotional experience associated with actual or potential tissue damage or described by the patient in terms of such damage". The definition of chronic pain is even more arbitrary: "pain that has persisted beyond normal tissue healing time (> 3 months)".

Treatment of acute pain focuses on its cause. Treatment or management of chronic pain focuses on the effects it is causing and is designed to limit disability and improve the patient's quality of life to the maximum, both socially and physically.

Classification is difficult and not helpful in formulating general principles of management. It is the severity of the chronic pain that affects patients, not the multiple causes or sites. The principle is to address chronic pain as a distinct diagnostic concept arising from any site or cause. This will help practical management in primary care.

Patients with chronic pain use primary care services up to five times more often than the general population. They are usually over-prescribed, over-investigated and over-referred, using up vast amounts of health care resources

Treatment or management of chronic pain focuses on the effects it is causing and is designed to limit disability and improve the patient's quality of life to the maximum, both socially and physically

Epidemiology of chronic pain

- Common problem. The World Health Organization (WHO) estimate that 22% of primary care attenders are sufferers.
- A UK population-based study estimated that the total prevalence (mild to severe) was 46%.
- Prevalence of severe, disabling, chronic pain is 5–10%.
- It is more common in older people.
- Lower socioeconomic groups have a higher incidence.
- Women are possibly at greater risk.
- Associated conditions are depression and poor social support.
- Recovery (unless diagnosed very early) seems to be rare.
- Management objectives need to be realistic.
- Preventative measures are important.

"The principle is to address chronic pain as a distinct diagnostic concept arising from any site or cause. This will help practical management in primary care"

Impact and ability to work

The experience of chronic pain may be subjective but the impact is wide ranging, causing disability (inability to live a normal life, tiredness, disturbed sleep patterns) and sometimes reduced earning capacity or even unemployment (Fig. 37). There is a loss of other physical and social roles and of hobbies and leisure pursuits. The effect on the family can be catastrophic, causing disharmony and social isolation for the patient and occasionally for the whole family. The patient's problems may affect other family members, leading to problems such as depression, loss of self-esteem, anxiety and sleep disturbance.

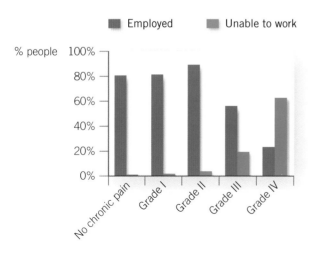

Fig. 37 Chronic pain severity and reported inability to work due to sickness or disability (people of employment age). Chronic pain reduces the ability to work, which makes the pain itself more severe. This graph shows how the percentage of people unable to work for health reasons is greater in people with severe chronic pain, reaching 60% at the most severe. Reprinted with kind permission of Blair Smith from **arc** In Practice 2002;9.

Primary care assessment and diagnosis

- Most patients with chronic pain have not discussed this diagnosis with their GP or been told that the diagnosis is chronic pain.
- The diagnosis needs to be made and discussed with the patient before progress can be made and pain management instigated.
- The diagnosis is not always readily accepted by the patient. A number of consultations may be necessary and the subject discussed from different angles.
- When dysfunctional disorders (see Fig. 40 page 78) are the underlying medical condition, discussion may take longer and more educational input will be required before the patient is "ready for change" (page 115).
- Some patients find difficulty in separating their medical condition (RA, OA) from their chronic pain. Medical personnel also have difficulty with this, assuming that the patient's medical condition is not well controlled.

> **❝** *Some patients find difficulty in separating their medical condition (RA, OA) from their chronic pain. Medical personnel also have difficulty with this, assuming that the patient's medical condition is not well controlled* **❞**

Management

Management must balance treatment and rehabilitation. It is important to have realistic goals for the individual that must be discussed with the patient, even if the goals change at a later date. This may include the patient returning to work (Fig. 37). It is equally important to discuss what cannot be cured. This concept is not new to primary care where medicine is based around "the individual" but it is harder to accept.

Drug treatment

For more details, see page 124. The WHO analgesic ladder (Fig. 38), developed for cancer pain, is applicable to most chronic pain cases. The Oxford Pain table should be consulted for alternative therapies (see appendix 5). Remember to use other team members:

Fig. 38 WHO analgesic ladder

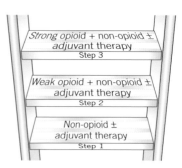

Strong opioid + non-opioid ± *adjuvant* therapy
Step 3

Weak opioid + non-opioid ± *adjuvant* therapy
Step 2

Non-opioid ± *adjuvant* therapy
Step 1

- Physiotherapy can offer more than merely the transcutaneous electrical nerve stimulation (TENS) machine.
- Occupational therapy (OT) can make a real difference, especially around the home.
- If available, counselling, preferably from a psychologist, can be helpful.
- Employment problems may require social service input as well as OT assessment for aids.
- Secondary care help may be needed for disease-modifying anti-rheumatic drugs (DMARDs) if there is RA, nerve blocks and surgical intervention.

Be judicious in the use of secondary care and tertiary referrals. Pain clinics may help but patients find more benefit from a good, understanding GP and a primary care team that is prepared to offer support and discuss things kindly and realistically.

Complementary medicine

Many patients attend a variety of therapists, often with apparent benefit. Some are virtually considered mainstream therapies, e.g., acupuncture and homeopathy. Some Primary Care Trusts (PCTs) have developed pain-management packs to help primary care staff manage patients in a structured way and to help with referral and management algorithms. Those produced by the Greater Glasgow NHS are excellent, including patient leaflets and questionnaires to help with patient management. Details of the following, or how to obtain them, are included in appendix 4:

- guidelines for management of pain,
- pain self-assessment chart,
- oswestry pain questionnaire,
- referral to Glasgow pain service,
- patient pain record (primary care),
- emotion questionnaire.

Fibromyalgia

The term fibromyalgia has been used since 1981. It is a diagnosis given to patients who have chronic pain (pain itself is the disorder), fatiguability and tender points (Fig. 39). It is probably best considered as affecting a specific group of patients within dysfunctional disorders: a group more easily defined as they have tender points. Dysfunctional disorders can be considered as a very broad spectrum of conditions and can be viewed as a continuum. All specialities in medicine deal with patients having dysfunctional disorders, such as those in Fig. 40.

> ❝ Be judicious in the use of secondary care and tertiary referrals. Pain clinics may help but patients find more benefit from a good, understanding GP and a primary care team that is prepared to offer support and discuss things kindly and realistically ❞

> ❝ Dysfunctional disorders can be considered as a very broad spectrum of conditions and can be viewed as a continuum. All specialities in medicine deal with patients having dysfunctional disorders ❞

Fig. 39 The cycle of pain and sleep disturbance. Reprinted from Fibromyalgia, **arc** patient information leaflet.

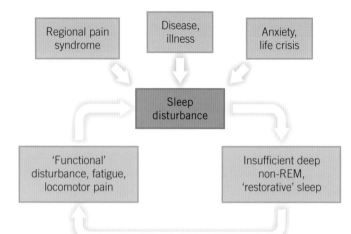

Fig. 40 Dysfunctional disorders

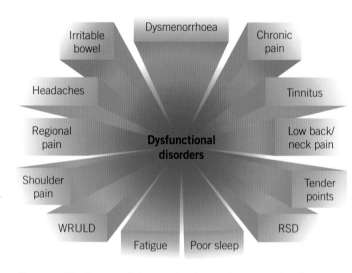

« The diagnosis is based on a history of chronic, widespread pain with the presence of at least 11 of 18 specified tender points. Fibromyalgia is not a distinct entity but is one end of a continuous spectrum »

Patients with these conditions tend to be overinvestigated and over-referred, looking for an organic cause.

Principal symptoms

In 1990, the American College of Rheumatology (ACR) published their criteria (Fig. 41), which are now internationally accepted. The diagnosis is based on a history of chronic, widespread pain with the presence of at least 11 of 18 specified tender points. Fibromyalgia is not a distinct entity but is one end of a continuous spectrum. Using the ACR criteria, the prevalence of chronic widespread pain is around 10% of the population.

Criterion	Definition
History of widespread pain	Pain is considered widespread when all of the following are present: pain in the left side of the body, pain in the right side of the body, pain above the waist, and pain below the waist. In addition, axial skeletal pain (cervical spine or anterior chest or thoracic spine or low back) must be present. In this definition, shoulder and buttock pain is considered as pain for each involved side. "Low back" pain is considered lower segment pain.
Pain in 11 of 18 tender point sites on digital palpation	Pain, on digital palpation, must be present in at least 11 of the following 18 tender point sites: **Occiput:** bilateral, at the suboccipital muscle insertions **Low cervical:** bilateral, at the anterior aspects of the intertransverse spaces at C5-C7 **Trapezius:** bilateral, at the midpoint of the upper border **Supraspinatus:** bilateral, at the origins, above the scapulae spine near the medial border **Second rib:** bilateral, at the second costochondral junctions, just lateral to the junctions on upper surfaces **Lateral epicondyle:** bilateral, 2 cm distal to the epicondyles **Gluteal:** bilateral, in outer quadrants of buttocks in anterior fold of muscle **Greater trochanter:** bilateral, posterior to the trochanteric prominence **Knee:** bilateral, at the medial fat pad proximal to the joint line Digital palpation should be performed with an approximate force of 4 kg. For a tender point to be considered "positive" the subject must state that the palpation was painful. "Tender" is not to be considered "painful".

Patients have fibromyalgia if both criteria are satisfied.
Widespread pain must have been present for ≥ 3 months.
The presence of a second clinical disorder does not exclude the diagnosis of fibromyalgia.

Fig. 41 The American College of Rheumatology 1990 criteria for the classification of fibromyalgia. The American College of Rheumatology 1990 Criteria for the Classification of Fibromyalgia. Report of the Multicenter Criteria Committee. Wolfe F, et al. *Arthritis Rheum* 1990;33:160-72. Reprinted by permission of Wiley-Liss, Inc., a subsidiary of John Wiley & Sons, Inc.

Other symptoms of fibromyalgia and associated problems
Pain
This is often aggravated by stress, cold and activity. It is often associated with generalized morning stiffness, often with subjective swelling of the extremities. For example, the patient may have the sensation that the fingers are grossly swollen but their appearance is normal or with possibly minimal swelling. There may also be paraesthesiae and dysaesthesiae of the hands and feet.

Fatiguability

This may be extreme and vary from day to day. It may occur after minimal exertion, even washing up.

Non-restorative sleep

- wakes unrefreshed,
- forgetful,
- poor concentration,
- diffuse abdominal pain and variable bowel habit,
- weepy,
- headaches (occipital, bi-frontal),
- urinary frequency: urgency day and night,
- low affect,
- dysmenorrhoea.

Fig. 42 Pathogenetic mechanisms in chronic widespread pain and fibromyalgia that are important for treatment strategies. Adapted with kind permission of Stefan Bergman from In Practice, **arc** 2003;10.

Pathogenesis of chronic widespread pain and fibromyalgia

Evidence is accumulating that peripheral factors interact with altered central nervous system processing of nociceptive stimuli (Fig. 42). Chronic widespread pain (CWP) can be present with other conditions (e.g., OA) but the pain is out of all proportion to the usual pain severity of the associated condition. Therefore the diagnosis is CWP rather than

Pathogenetic mechanisms in chronic widespread pain and fibromyalgia that are important for treatment strategies	
Peripheral pain generator	Traumatic tissue damage Osteoarthritis Inflammatory rheumatic diseases Muscular tension Disc herniation Endometriosis Migraine
Peripheral sensitization	More responsive nociceptors
Central sensitization and disinhibition	Facilitated transmission of pain signals
Cognitive processes	Thoughts and memories
Emotional processes	Anxiety and depression
Stress and psychosocial situation	
Behaviour	Avoidance and immobilization Withdrawal and escape Muscle contraction

knee OA. It also explains why, when these patients undergo an operation, there is a greater risk of a poor result or a return of pain within a short timeframe. An example of this is inappropriate back surgery.

Peripheral tissue nociceptors are normally silent unless there are noxious stimuli. In order for CWP to develop, the nociceptors must become sensitized, producing an enhanced response that can be noxious or non-noxious (Fig. 43). They may also discharge spontaneously. These stimuli are relayed via the dorsal horn and spinothalamic tract to the thalamus and higher centres. As with all transmissions, there are descending inhibitory signals that are also influenced by endorphins and serotonin. These inhibitory influences may be reduced so that there is now a problematic pain situation caused by peripheral sensitization, central sensitization and diminished central inhibition. Stress appears to be able to disturb the normal hypothalamus–pituitary–adrenal axis. Patients with fibromyalgia (CWP), low back pain and chronic fatigue have been shown to have this disturbance. In addition, neurohormonal system changes interact with central pain perception. Lastly, there are the psychological components (attention, cognition, emotions, behavioural changes), each of which will have a different influence on the individual patient, depending on the time course and associated diagnoses (Fig. 44).

> *Peripheral tissue nociceptors are normally silent unless there are noxious stimuli. In order for CWP to develop, the nociceptors must become sensitized, producing an enhanced response that can be noxious or non-noxious*

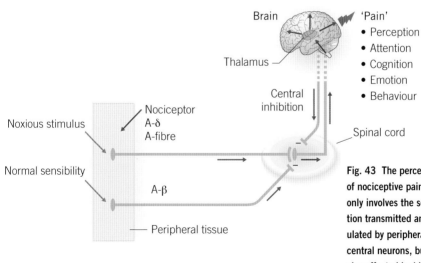

Fig. 43 The perception of nociceptive pain not only involves the sensation transmitted and regulated by peripheral and central neurons, but is also affected by higher brain function. Reprinted with kind permission of Stefan Bergman from In Practice, **arc** 2003;10.

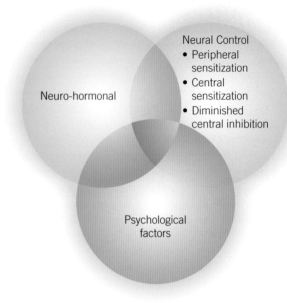

Neural Control
- Peripheral sensitization
- Central sensitization
- Diminished central inhibition

Neuro-hormonal

Psychological factors

Fig. 44 Interaction of the control mechanisms leading to the occurrence of chronic widespread pain

Risk factors

CWP is more likely to develop in patients with long-standing regional pain. Patients move within this pain spectrum but those with higher tender-point counts tend to be at the severe end of the spectrum. Other factors have been discussed under the epidemiology of chronic pain (page 74).

Practical management

Fig. 45 provides a practical approach to assessment and treatment of patients with musculoskeletal pain from a GP's point of view.

Regional pain or non-widespread pain

Regional pain or non-widespread pain is at the other end of the spectrum/continuum of widespread pain or fibromyalgia. Good examples are chronic low back pain and chronic shoulder pain. Historically, these conditions have been poorly managed. Today's practical management options have been discussed under back pain, neck pain, chronic pain and fibromyalgia. The important principles are management of pain and self-management. Fig. 45 is also helpful, as individual patients will have different contributions of these three components and so management strategies will vary accordingly.

❝ Regional pain or non–widespread pain is at the other end of the spectrum/ continuum of widespread pain or fibromyalgia. Good examples are chronic low back pain and chronic shoulder pain ❞

A practical approach to assessment and treatment of patients with musculoskeletal pain from a GP's point of view

Believe the patient's experience and description of pain
Do a thorough clinical examination at the first visit
Treat acute pain adequately
Search for peripheral pain generators
Pay attention to cognitive factors
Pay attention to emotional factors
Pay attention to stress and psychosocial factors
Pay attention to central sensitization and central disinhibition
Encourage physical exercise
Massage therapy, acupuncture and TENS could be adjuvant
Consider cognitive behavioural therapy
Educate and motivate the patient
Create a multidisciplinary team, perhaps in your Primary Care Trust

Fig. 45 A practical approach to assessment and treatment of patients with musculoskeletal pain from a GP's point of view. Adapted with kind permission of Stefan Bergman from **arc** In Practice, 2003;10.

Hypermobility

This is a common, normal variant at the opposite end of the mobility spectrum from restriction of movement. Mobility varies with race, age, hormones, environment and activity; gymnasts and ballet dancers are more flexible.

Clinical presentation

* Hypermobility can be generalized, affecting all joints including the spine, or more localized.
* Hypermobility may be localized, affecting:
  - peripheral joints,
  - spine,
  - upper body,
  - lower body,
  - one side of the body.
* Patients with lax joints tend to suffer more joint and tendon problems than the average person.
* Check for hypermobility in any patient presenting with a musculoskeletal problem at any age.
* Females often present with joint problems relating to hypermobility within 3 years of the menopause.

" Check for hypermobility in any patient presenting with a musculoskeletal problem at any age "

83

- Other patients present within 3 years of ceasing athletic activities or when taking up activities again.
- Adolescents with anterior knee pain and genu recurvatum invariably have hypermobility as the underlying condition. The scenario appears to be loss of quadriceps power to protect against overextension of the joint, leading to bruising of the articular cartilage and, in the most severe cases, joint effusion.

§§ Classically, in adolescents, anterior knee pain presents within 3 years of the menarche, puberty or when there is a major growth spurt §§

- Classically, in adolescents, anterior knee pain presents within 3 years of the menarche or puberty or when there is a major growth spurt.
- The classical scoring system is the Beighton Score (Fig. 46). Patients who have a full score can usually do contortionist acts but patients with more localized hypermobility are not uncommon and benefit from an understanding consultation.

Treatment and management

- The treatment is around physical therapies: the patient should wear trainers or use sorbothane arch supports, accompanied by quality physiotherapy and exercises to develop the quadriceps to help protect the joint.
- Patients with severe anterior knee pain can be helped by removing 2–3cm off the heel of a pair of trainers and then gluing on a thin replacement heel so that the heels are lower than normal. The "bruised" cartilage will take weeks to settle.
- The surgical procedure of a lateral release should be reserved for patients who do not have hypermobility otherwise there is a major risk of converting anterior knee pain into a permanently deficient joint and associated loss of athletic activities.

Fig. 46 Hypermobility scoring: Beighton scores

	Right side	Left side
Dorsiflexion of the 5th metacarpophalangeal joint to 90°	1	1
Apposition of the thumb to volar aspect of forearm	1	1
Hyperextension of the elbow by ≥ 10°	1	1
Hyperextension of the knee by ≥ 10°	1	1
Hands flat on the floor with knees extended		1
Total	9 points	

- Sports personnel with hypermobility must be encouraged to warm up and, more importantly, warm down, as they appear to have greater stiffness following exercise than the average. Warming down and stretching exercises limit arthralgia and myalgia. Stretching exercises performed for a few minutes every hour for 2–4 hours following exercise are beneficial: they greatly limit the stiffness experienced the next morning. Warming down is the answer, not giving up the sporting activity.

Musculoskeletal problems in children and teenagers and the active elderly

Most lower limb problems in children and teenagers, aged 2–20 years, are within the range of normality and reassurance that all will be well is required. Quite often there will be a third presence during the consultation of a teacher, social worker or work associate who is concerned about the child. The normal age range at which children begin to walk varies from 8 months to 4 years. Some children walk on their toes for months; check for any shoe problems that may impede progress. Most children walk abnormally at some time but most adults walk normally!

Flat feet

These are normal in children as the medial arch develops within 2–3 years of walking. Hypermobile children have flat feet but an arch will appear if they stand on tiptoe. Check that there are no tight bands or fixed deformities as these may require an expert opinion.

In-toe/out-toe gait, squinting patellae, knock knees and bow legs

- In-toe gait usually resolves of its own accord by the age of 8–9 years. It may be caused by misshapen feet with medial or varus displacement of the metatarsals, excessive internal tibial torsion or persistent femoral anteversion. Treat expectantly.
- Out-toe gait is common and often familial. Treat expectantly.
- Persistent femoral anteversion (bilateral squinting patellae) occurs when the femoral head and neck point in the same direction as the patellae. It is normal in babies and, where it persists, should resolve by 8 years old. Squinting patellae is the result of internal rotation of the femur to keep the head in the acetabulum. Expert opinion, and possibly surgery, may be required for patients with squinting patellae plus cerebral palsy or similar pathology.
- Children are usually bow legged (genu varus) until they reach 2 years; few require expert advice. Most children drift from genu varus at 2 years old to genu valgus (knock knees) at around 7 years.

❝Sports personnel with hypermobility must be encouraged to warm up and, more importantly, warm down, as they appear to have greater stiffness following exercise than the average❞

❝Most children walk abnormally at some time but most adults walk normally❞

> **If the child is under 6 years old and there is less than 6cm between the knees (bow legs) or less than 6cm between the ankles (knock knees), the situation will probably be self-limiting**

> **If uncertain, see the patient again after 6 weeks and then follow up every 6 months and refer where appropriate**

If genu valgus persists in older children, referral may be required but surgery should be deferred for as long as possible.

Rule of six

If the child is under 6 years old and there is less than 6cm between the knees (bow legs) or less than 6cm between the ankles (knock knees), the situation will probably be self-limiting. If uncertain, see the patient again after 6 weeks and then follow up every 6 months and refer where appropriate. Consider referral/expert opinion if:

- the family requires more reassurance,
- joints appear to have a limited range of movement,
- there is uneven growth in the lower limbs,
- contracture deformities are developing or present,
- the temperature of the two limbs is different,
- there is an associated pathology, e.g., cerebral palsy.

Nocturnal idiopathic musculoskeletal pain syndrome: growing pains

- Occurs in the lower limbs at 4–12 years old, most common at 10–12 years, and affects 4% of all children.
- In older children, pain has often been present for some time before they are seen by a doctor.
- More common in active children and may be present after exercise during the day.
- May cause disturbed nights, poor sleeping and crying at night. Sometimes abdominal pain and headaches occur.
- Often stress factors at school, bullying, domestic problems and lack of friends.

Treatment

- reassurance,
- encourage self-massage/rubbing of limb,
- paracetamol can be taken if necessary; NSAIDs are rarely required.

Differential diagnosis

> **If the child has a limp, growing pains can be excluded**

Few conditions mimic growing pains. The history and examination (which should be normal) will exclude juvenile chronic arthritis, leukaemia, bone trauma and infection. If the child has a limp, growing pains can be excluded.

Osteoid osteoma

This is a rare benign tumour that is difficult to differentiate from growing pains. Pain is less localized, primarily nocturnal and often relieved dramatically by NSAIDs. It becomes more permanent and is not relieved by rest. Computed tomography (CT) scan will show abnormalities earlier than an X-ray. Secondary care referral is mandatory.

Non-accidental injury

Do not forget to consider this possibility. The following should ring alarm bells:

- frequent surgery or clinic attendances,
- behavioural problems,
- odd or suspicious family dynamics,
- frequent reports from the hospital casualty department,
- multiple bruises, often spontaneous, especially cigar-shaped bruises,
- haemarthrosis not due to a bleeding problem,
- brown induration over the hands and knuckles,
- child refuses to bear weight, often accompanied by a joint effusion,
- skin lesions difficult to diagnose,
- bone chips on X-rays,
- previous fractures on X-ray, especially if they involve uncommon fracture sites.

Irritable hip/toxic synovitis

- Commonest cause of a limp in children, particularly in boys aged 3–10 years.
- Most can be treated at home with bedrest and paracetamol. If problem has not resolved within 3 days, expert advice must be sought.
- If the patient has a fever, admission to hospital is necessary. If the temperature is > 38°C and the ESR > 20mm/h, consider osteomyelitis or hip sepsis. Ultrasound may be useful in detecting an effusion and helping to decide the differential diagnosis.
- Irritable hip may present as knee pain.

Legg-Perthes' disease (ischaemic necrosis of the femoral head)

- Boy:girl ratio of 8:1 is of no practical value when there is only one patient with this complaint. Peak onset age is 4–6 years.
- More common in children who are small for their age with small feet, suggesting that it might be linked to growth problems. It is caused by a mismatch between the femoral head growth plate and the penetrating blood vessels. Blood vessels become blocked, producing ischaemic necrosis.
- Child may present with non-localized pain or pain in the knee but usually with a limp, with or without pain.
- Second hip presents within 3 years in 10–20% of cases.

❝Legg-Perthes' disease more common in children who are small for their age with small feet, suggesting that it might be linked to growth problems. It is caused by a mismatch between the femoral head growth plate and the penetrating blood vessels. Blood vessels become blocked, producing ischaemic necrosis❞

- Younger patients do better and usually only require monitoring with restricted sports activities. Overall, 40% of patients only require monitoring.
- Older patients usually require some form of containment of the femoral head within the acetabulum and await repair/revascularization: 60% of all patients require this approach. Containment is either surgical or requires the use of braces.
- Psychological effects on the child and parents can be immense.

Adolescents and activity-related problems

Fig. 47 outlines the common, likely and less common problems associated with activity in adolescents.

Fig. 47 Adolescents and activity-related problems. Reprinted from the University of Bath Diploma, Module 5 – Lower Limb.

Snapping hip

Common in runners, the snapping noise (also palpable) is caused by the iliotibial band slipping over the greater trochanter. The patient will usually seek help when/if pain develops from a trochanteric bursitis.

	Likely/common	Less common
Hip and groin problems	Muscular problems such as groin strains or groin pain Tendon problems Bursitis Slipped femoral epiphysis	Avascular necrosis of the femoral head, e.g., from use of steroids Psoriatic arthritis Juvenile chronic arthritis Consequences of Legg-Perthes' disease Tumours
Knee problems	Jumper's knee Cartilage/meniscal problems Knee effusions ± haemarthrosis Osgood-Schlatter disease Anterior knee pain/hypermobility Other activity related knee problems, e.g., twisted knee Runner's knee Achilles tendonitis	Recurrent dislocation of the patellae/patella tracking problems Osteochondritis dissecans
Lower leg problems	Achilles bursitis Other activity related problems, e.g., bruising of calf and other muscle strains/sprains Viral aches and pains Shin splints	Stress factors Compartmental problems Haematological problems, e.g., haemophilia, leukaemia Bacterial infections – septicaemia causes stiff and painful movement of most joints Tumours of the bones Pain crisis from sickle cell disease
Ankle and foot problems	Twisted ankle/sprained ankle Other sprains of the foot tendons, joints Plantar fasciitis Extensor tendon problems	Metatarsalgia Stress fractures Flat feet Bursitis

Slipped femoral epiphysis (causing injury to the growth zone)

This is classically seen in boys, but rare enough in primary care that the diagnosis has to be considered in either sex if an adolescent presents with hip pain or pain referred to the knee. Influential factors are trauma and hormonal changes and many of these patients are overweight. The pain can be in the groin or the knee and weight bearing may be impossible. If slippage is slow/gradual, the diagnosis is harder to suspect. On examination, hip rotation and abduction will be limited. X-ray will confirm the diagnosis and orthopaedic referral is mandatory.

Groin strain

- Painful and common. Usually a clear history of cause and provoking factors.
- Most common in young athletes who do not warm up properly or who overuse their adductors (Fig. 17, page 39).
- Pain localized to one area on the pubic bone.
- Pain reproduced by pressing legs inwards against resistance whilst lying flat on the examination couch.
- Differential diagnosis: hip disease, hernias, testicular problems.

Shin splints (medial tibial syndrome)

- an overuse injury,
- seen in intensively trained sports personnel, especially if they change surfaces, shoes and technique for each surface,
- pain, tenderness and sometimes swelling experienced on lower medial margin of one or both tibia (Fig. 48),

> *This is classically seen in boys, but rare enough in primary care that the diagnosis has to be considered in either sex if an adolescent presents with hip pain or pain referred to the knee. Influential factors are trauma and hormonal changes and many of these patients are overweight*

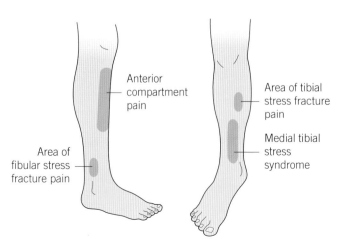

Anterior compartment pain

Area of tibial stress fracture pain

Medial tibial stress syndrome

Area of fibular stress fracture pain

Fig. 48 Areas of stress fracture pain, shin splints and anterior compartment pain. Reprinted from the University of Bath Diploma, Module 5 – Lower Limb.

89

- pain initially only when exercising but as it progresses, pain present even on cessation of activity,
- differential diagnosis: stress/fatigue fractures, which are much more painful, and compartment syndromes.

Stress fractures of the tibia and fibula
- Usually occur in the upper two-thirds of the tibia with marked tenderness and swelling.
- Fibula stress fractures are usually within 7cm of the lateral malleolus with similar signs and symptoms.
- The most useful investigation is an isotope bone scan (X-ray will be normal in the acute stages; fracture line usually only shows as healing occurs).

Compartment syndromes
Activity must be encouraged. Generally, adolescents and young adults will take most injuries in their stride. Active older people, especially those who were inactive in their youth, are more prone to injury, take badly to the "inconvenience" and recover more slowly.

This is a common problem for the active elderly. It is an overuse injury caused by too much walking or hiking, resulting pain in the anterior or posterior compartments of the lower leg. There are more problems with the anterior compartment because it is smaller and more rigidly bound. Activity causes the muscles to swell and pain results. The pain may be diffuse or localized and usually subsides on standing still for a few minutes. The usual treatment is rest and limitation of walking activities. In the over-65s, NSAIDs/Cox-2s taken before activity should help. Surgical division of the fascia is rarely required.

Rheumatoid arthritis

RA is an inflammatory, symmetrical polyarthritis that is chronic and persistent and leads to loss of function and increased mortality. It is three times more common in women than in men. The diagnostic criteria for RA are given in appendix 3.

Aetiology and pathogenesis
The aetiology of RA is unknown although infectious agents of various kinds have been proposed. RA is believed to be an autoimmune disease triggered by unknown autoantigens. Hormonal factors may be important and may explain the female preponderance and the dramatic improvement in disease activity in many women during pregnancy with a return of disease after delivery.

"RA is an inflammatory, symmetrical polyarthritis that is chronic and persistent and leads to loss of function and increased mortality. It is three times more common in women than in men"

The pathogenesis is better understood. RA is strongly linked to human leukocyte antigen DR4 (HLADR4), which is carried on the surface of macrophages and antigen-presenting cells. HLADR4 molecules present antigens to T-cells, which activates the T-cells, enabling them to initiate a cascade of immune and inflammatory mechanisms. The histology of the rheumatoid synovial membrane shows many activated T-cells as well as the presence of antigen-presenting cells bearing HLADR4 on their surface. Thus, there is abundant direct and indirect evidence that T-cells maintain inflammation in the rheumatoid synovium. Macrophages that release a number of inflammatory mediators, including human tumour necrosis factor alpha (TNFα) and interleukin 1 (IL-1), contribute to the inflammatory changes. Inhibition of TNFα and IL-1 using biologic agents demonstrate that TNFα and IL-1 are directly involved in the pathogenesis of RA. Activation of synovial membrane fibroblasts leads to the release of enzymes that cause cartilage degradation and activation of osteoclasts then leads to the characteristic bony erosions seen on X-rays.

The B-lymphocytes are also importantly involved in the pathogenesis of RA. First, B-cells carry HLADR4 on their surface and may act as antigen-presenting cells, stimulating T-cells. Second, T-cells, once activated, activate B-cells, which then secrete immunoglobulins including RF. RF can form immune complexes and activate complement and macrophages, thereby contributing to synovial inflammation. Thus, RF is not only a useful diagnostic tool but is a central element in the pathogenesis of the disease.

Presentation

History

RA may have three types of presentation:

- The more characteristic presentation is that of an insidious inflammatory arthritis characterized by pain in the joints, early morning stiffness lasting > 45 minutes, frequent nocturnal waking, swelling of the joints and tenderness on palpation or movement.
- A minority of patients may present extremely acutely with an inflammatory polyarthritis.
- RA may occasionally present in elderly patients with a picture that is very similar to PMR.

Patients frequently complain of being generally unwell, have fatigue that may be extreme, and may have reduced appetite with weight loss. Fever is unusual.

❝ The more characteristic presentation is that of an insidious inflammatory arthritis characterized by pain in the joints, early morning stiffness lasting > 45 minutes, frequent nocturnal waking, swelling of the joints and tenderness on palpation or movement ❞

> *Non-specific agglutination tests for RF such as the latex test are too sensitive and not sufficiently specific; referral of patients in whom only the latex test is positive should be discouraged; more specific tests, such as the newer agglutination test or the Rose-Waaler test, should be used*

Examination

The clinical examination shows inflammatory swelling of the joints: joints are swollen, hot, tender on palpation and painful on passive and active movement. The skin is rarely discoloured, which is a useful distinguishing characteristic from crystal arthritis and infective arthritis.

- There may be nodules on the extensor surfaces, particularly of the elbows, but this is a rare presenting feature today.
- Polyarthritis must involve at least three large joint groups, e.g., wrists, MCP joints or proximal interphalangeal (PIP) joints. The symmetry need not involve the identical joints in each of these groups.
- There are no associated physical findings on clinical examination although there may occasionally be splenomegaly and lymphadenopathy. There is no characteristic skin rash.

Differential diagnosis

An established case of RA is unmistakable. The problem arises in diagnosis of an early case. Under these circumstances, RA could be confused with several diseases including peripheral arthropathy of the spondyloarthritides. However, the passage of time soon dispels this.

- Occasionally, acute viral arthritides may present with a polyarthritis but they do not persist long enough to enter the differential diagnosis.
- Polyarticular psoriatic arthritis should not cause any confusion but there may be a family history of psoriasis in first-degree relatives without the patient exhibiting the disease.

Investigations

These investigations should be carried out in primary care:

- ESR and CRP (elevated),
- RF (positive, but frequency of RF positivity is low in early-stage disease),
- red flag: non-specific agglutination tests for RF such as the latex test are too sensitive and not sufficiently specific; referral of patients in whom only the latex test is positive should be discouraged; more specific tests, such as the newer agglutination test or the Rose-Waaler test, should be used,
- increasingly, anti-CCP (antibody to cyclic, citrullinated peptides) will be used as this autoantibody may be more specific and sensitive for the diagnosis of RA,
- normochromic normocytic anaemia (frequent), the anaemia of inflammatory disease,
- white cells (usually no disturbance, although occasionally low neutrophils as part of Felty's syndrome: neutropenia, RA, high RF titres and leg ulcers),

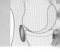

- radiological examination of hands and feet (may show erosions); erosions first appear in the feet, in early cases, there may be only periarticular osteoporosis without erosions.

Assuming that the appropriate investigations have been carried out in primary care, secondary care can use newer diagnostic imaging techniques to diagnose early erosions. This is particularly true for the use of high-resolution ultrasonography.

Management

Optimum management of RA requires a multi-disciplinary team consisting of a rheumatologist, a nurse practitioner, a physiotherapist, an occupational therapist and other support staff such as a chiropodist and, unfortunately, an orthopaedic surgeon in advanced disease with major joint damage. The GP is an integral part of this team and should be involved in long-term follow-up and management of the patient with RA on the basis of shared care protocols.

Patient education

From the beginning, the patient must be educated about the nature of the disease, the importance of controlling inflammation and the nature of the drugs they are to receive and their possible side effects. Patients should be given either in-house publications or publications from sources such as the Arthritis Research Campaign (**arc**) or patient support groups.

Pain control

A survey of patients by the National RA Society (NRAS) showed that one of the most important needs of patients with RA was adequate pain control. Pain control can be achieved using NSAIDs or Cox-2s. Pure analgesics can also be used but these are not generally as effective. The best pain control is achieved by adequate and maximal control of inflammation. In joints that have a large degree of secondary OA from chronic destruction, pain may be due to OA rather than ongoing inflammation.

Inflammation control

The control of inflammation can be achieved in two ways: DMARDs and biologics.

- The DMARDs include methotrexate, sulphasalazine, gold salts, antimalarials, cyclosporine, azathioprine and leflunomide (appendix 1). The most commonly used drugs are sulphasalazine and methotrexate. Their use has been validated by properly conducted RCTs. Leflunomide has been shown to be at least as effective as sulphasalazine and methotrexate with few serious side effects (Fig. 49), although about 20% of patients may suffer from diarrhoea.

“Increasingly, anti-CCP will be used as this autoantibody may be more specific and sensitive for diagnosis of RA”

93

Fig. 49 Response rates with leflunomide versus other DMARDs, expressed as the American College of Rheumatology criteria based on a 20%, 50% or 70% improvement in a number of parameters, including swollen and tender joint counts, global scores and C-reative protein.
Reprinted from Smolen et al, *Lancet* 1999;353:259 with permission from Elsevier (a) and Strand V, et al. *Arch Intern Med* 1999;159:2542. Copyrighted © 1999, American Medical Association. All rights reserved (b).

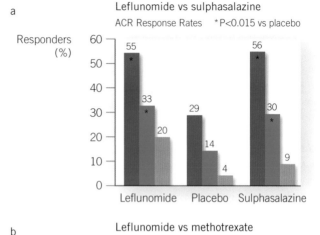

a

Leflunomide vs sulphasalazine
ACR Response Rates   *P<0.015 vs placebo

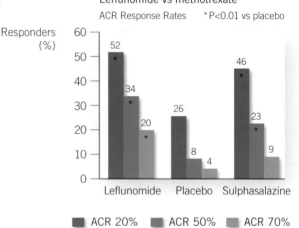

b

Leflunomide vs methotrexate
ACR Response Rates   *P<0.01 vs placebo

ACR 20%   ACR 50%   ACR 70%

- DMARDs can also be used in combination therapies, some of which have been subjected to RCTs. Both single and combination DMARD therapy is prescribed in secondary care.
- Treatment with biologics. The National Institute for Clinical Excellence (NICE) has laid down criteria for the use of biologics for treatment-resistant RA: failure to respond to two or more DMARDs, either because of lack of efficacy or because of toxicity, and a Disease Activity Score (DAS) of more than 5.1. The DAS is an objective measure of clinical activity. There are currently three anti-TNF therapies available: etanercept, infliximab and adalimumab. An IL-1 receptor antagonist, anakinra (Kineret), is self-administered subcutaneously by patients daily.

Surgery

Unfortunately, there is still a very high rate of surgical intervention in patients with RA. It is hoped that the present policy of early diagnosis and early institution of aggressive and effective therapy to limit inflammation will render surgery less likely in the future. There should be optimum collaboration between the rheumatologist, orthopaedic surgeon, GP and patient for effective delivery of surgical therapy. The ideal situation is early rather than late referral.

TNF therapy

In RA, targeted therapies directed against TNFα have produced great benefit to patients who have failed more than two DMARDs.
There are three such targeted therapies:
- Infliximab (Remicade) is a monoclonal antibody, partly human and partly mouse. It is given by intravenous infusion every 8 weeks.
- Etanercept (Enbrel) is a construct consisting of the TNFα receptor linked to the Fc fragment of immunoglobulin G (IgG). It is given by the patient subcutaneously twice a week.
- Adalimumab (Humira), a fully human anti-TNF monoclonal antibody, is self-administered subcutaneously by the patient once every 2 weeks.

Etanercept and adalimumab are more convenient than infliximab because they can be administered by the patient subcutaneously and patients do not have to attend hospital for intravenous infusions. With increasing familiarity with the use of these biologics, primary care physicians may be involved in their long-term supervision in partnership with the rheumatologist. In future, targeted therapies may be delivered by orally active low-molecular-weight drugs – the DMARDs of the future.

Follow-up and prognosis
Follow-up

Since RA is a chronic persistent disease, follow-up is necessary both in primary and secondary care. This should be done on the basis of shared protocols agreed either locally or by the implementation of nationally agreed guidelines. With effective therapy, patients should see the rheumatologist at infrequent intervals of several months. Either the hospital or GP surgery can monitor for blood and other toxicities; results should be reviewed by both the GP and rheumatologist.
- An ideal situation is a hotline through which the patient or GP can access the secondary care centre. This should be manned by a nurse practitioner with adequate training in this area. For more obvious medical emergencies, medical staff should be approached.

❝Since RA is a chronic persistent disease, follow-up is necessary both in primary and secondary care. This should be done on the basis of shared protocols agreed either locally or by the implementation of nationally agreed guidelines❞

Prognosis

The prognosis for RA is not good. Not only is there high morbidity and increased mortality, but patients also have a high degree of social isolation with divorce and loss of work. It is hoped that the newer treatments will make a substantial and important difference to the outcome and ensuing quality of life. There is already evidence that good control of disease activity with methotrexate leads to a halving of the increased mortality. Adequate use of DMARDs can slow the rate of progression of erosive disease. Anti-TNF biologics have shown very impressive slowing of erosions and even cessation of erosions in RCTs. Whether this will be achieved in clinical practice is not yet clear. Such trials are relatively short term compared to the lifetime of the disease. Nevertheless, there is general optimism that the prognosis for patients with RA will be greatly transformed with better quality of life, less social isolation, more patients at work and fewer surgical interventions.

Diagnostic advances

Diagnosis of musculoskeletal diseases will be vastly improved by better and more widely available imaging technologies but the biggest impact will be in the realm of biochemical, immunological and genetic diagnostic methodologies. What follows is a brief overview of a rapidly expanding field. More details can be found on the Internet.

Biochemical methods

It is now possible to characterize even complex biological fluids with techniques such as two-dimensional gel electrophoresis and computer analysis to diagnose individual diseases, predict prognosis or even assess disease activity. In future, it may be possible to order such an investigation from appropriate primary care guidelines.

Immunological methods

The identification of new antigen/antibody systems that confer greater sensitivity and specificity for diagnosis of individual diseases is more exciting

Although autoantibodies have been used to diagnose rheumatic diseases for over 50 years, their systematic application in specific and disease-sensitive diagnostic algorithms is only now being developed. The identification of new antigen/antibody systems that confer greater sensitivity and specificity for diagnosis of individual diseases is more exciting. One such autoantibody, anti-CCP, has been identified for RA. Arginine, a constituent amino acid of protein molecules, can be citrullinated by peptidyl arginine deiminase. Proteins containing such modified arginines act as rheumatoid autoantigens. This autoantibody test is not yet available in primary care and is used in only a few secondary centres. Its more widespread use will increase the accuracy of RA diagnosis. It is hoped that this will have two important consequences: fewer referrals of patients with purported RA for a consultant opinion, and anti-CCP-positive patients seen by the rheumatologist as a matter of extreme urgency.

Genetic advances

There are two aspects to genetic diagnoses. The first is the use of germ line genetic differences to predict individuals at risk of developing a particular disease. Since the overwhelming majority of rheumatic diseases have a very large environmental component, this approach seems to have little clinical diagnostic utility. The one exception is to predict the toxic side effects of drugs when such effects are based on single-gene mutations. Measuring thiopurine methyltransferase levels in red blood cell can predict individuals at risk of serious haematological complications from azathioprine. The second is to measure the genes that are actively being transcribed in a particular tissue. Active genes in the synovial membrane in a patient presenting with RA could predict those individuals liable to have severe erosive disease and who should be treated more aggressively. Furthermore, expressed genes may also determine which individuals will respond to a particular therapy. These developments will deliver treatments tailored to individuals – maximizing benefit while minimizing toxicity.

> ❝ *Active genes in the synovial membrane in a patient presenting with RA could predict those individuals liable to have severe erosive disease* ❞

Crystal arthritis

The only two crystal arthritides that need to be considered are gout and pseudogout.

Gout

Gout is usually an acute monoarthritis presenting with inflammation that resolves within a few days.

> ❝ *Gout is usually an acute monoarthritis presenting with inflammation that resolves within a few days* ❞

Aetiology and pathogenesis

The solubility of uric acid is rather low. Excess uric acid in the blood leads to deposition of uric acid as crystals within joints and extra-articularly. This deposition leads to inflammation through the release of a number of inflammatory mediators including TNFα, IL-1 and prostaglandins. The mechanism of the hyperuricaemia is varied and may include:

- overproduction of uric acid,
- decreased excretion of uric acid by the kidney either idiopathically or through renal disease,
- prescription of diuretics that inhibit tubular uric acid excretion (e.g., thiazides),
- high purine intake, especially via beer.

Presentation

The patient presents with acute pain, tenderness and swelling over the involved joint. The pain is severe and lasts for several days but never more than 1 week.

- Classically, the MTP joint of the left big toe is involved, although any joint may be involved.
- Foot joints are more commonly affected.
- Skin over the involved joint may be red and may desquamate.

Clinical examination

The clinical examination shows all the signs of acute inflammation in the joint.

- Examination is difficult because of the extreme tenderness of the joint
- There may be extra-articular deposits of uric acid crystals known as tophi, particularly in sites such as the ears and over extensive surfaces of the body such as the elbow and knees.
- The patient may be obese.

Differential diagnosis

❝ Two differential diagnoses need to be entertained: infection of the joint and pseudogout ❞

Two differential diagnoses need to be entertained: infection of the joint and pseudogout. An infected joint may have all the characteristics of an acute gouty joint although the symptoms of pain and tenderness are never as extreme. There may be fever both in gout and in septic arthritis. As a rule, septic arthritis does not resolve after a few days. Pseudogout may also present in a similar manner to gout but may have a more insidious onset, particularly in the elderly patient, and the attacks usually persist for longer. The sites of predilection are different with pseudogout preferentially attacking the knees rather than small foot joints.

Investigations

In primary care:

- Estimate of serum uric acid levels to establish the diagnosis; demonstration of uric acid crystals within neutrophils in the synovial fluid is the diagnostic gold standard.

❝ Uric acid levels may fall to normal during an acute attack because of precipitation within tissues ❞

- Caution should be exercised in interpreting the results since uric acid levels may fall to normal during an acute attack because of precipitation within tissues.
- A full blood count, including ESR and CRP, will reveal neutrophil leukocytosis and elevated acute-phase response.
- If possible, synovial fluid or tissue fluid should be aspirated and rapidly sent to the nearest laboratory for birefringence polarizing microscopy to detect intracellular uric acid crystals and for

bacteriological examination for infection. Failing that, the patient should be sent as a matter of urgency to the nearest centre where these investigations can be done.

- The affected joint should be X-rayed to detect the punched-out erosions of gout or the chondrocalcinosis of pseudogout.

The rheumatologist may have more experience and expertise in aspirating joints for crystal examination. More elegant imaging techniques are not usually indicated in the diagnosis of gout.

The acute attack

- The acute attack is managed mainly using NSAIDs or, increasingly, Cox-2s because of their reduced gastrointestinal side effects. The choice of drug is a matter of individual preference and experience.
- Colchicine is not used to treat acute gout, because of the closeness of the therapeutic/toxic ratio, unless other anti-inflammatory drugs are contraindicated.

Long-term therapy

Some effort should be made to restrict dietary uric acid intake, particularly in beer. If diuretics are being used, their use should be revised and alternative treatments considered. The standby treatment is allopurinol. Allopurinol ($\leq$ 300mg single dose) should be used to reduce serum uric acid levels to well within normal. Given time, most tophi regress. There is a possibility of an acute gouty attack in the early stages of allopurinol therapy, which can be prevented by giving an NSAID or Cox-2 during the first month of allopurinol therapy.

> *Allopurinol ($\leq$ 300mg single dose) should be used to reduce serum uric acid levels to well within normal*

Follow-up and prognosis

Patients with gout should be followed up frequently if there is an alcohol problem for encouragement to desist. Uric acid needs to be monitored annually once it has stabilized within the normal range. Hyperuricaemia accompanies the metabolic syndrome characterized by central obesity, hypertension and maturity-onset diabetes. Patients should be screened for these conditions and appropriate measures taken. Well-controlled hyperuricaemia has an excellent prognosis.

Seronegative spondyloarthropathies

The seronegative spondyloarthropathies are a heterogeneous collection of diseases with ankylosing spondylitis as the prime example. They also include the spondylitis found in association with psoriasis, inflammatory bowel disease and reactive arthritis. One common link is the possession to a variable degree of the tissue-typing antigen, HLA-B27, which is associated with the spondylitis and not the arthritis.

Ankylosing spondylitis

Ankylosing spondylitis is an inflammatory disease of the spine that mainly affects young men and leads to progressive loss of spinal mobility with eventual bony ankylosis.

Aetiology and pathogenesis

The aetiology of ankylosing spondylitis is not known but it may be due to a bacterial infection of the gut. Some 95% of individuals with the disease are HLA-B27 positive, while the prevalence of this tissue type in the British population is around 8%. The disease is characterized by inflammation at three principal sites:

- apophyseal joints of the spine, leading to fibrous and eventually to bony ankylosis; hence, the name of the disease,
- enthesis (peripheral sites where ligaments or tendons attach to bone), which gives rise to enthesopathies, the most common of which occurs at the attachment of the tendoachilles or plantar fascia to the calcaneus,
- peripheral synovial joints, where there may be synovitis and even frank effusion.

The inflammation in both the spine and enthesis is characterized by the presence of inflammatory cells (neutrophils, mononuclear cells) and inflammatory cytokines (TNFα, IL-1). On histology, the synovial membrane cannot be distinguished from the synovitis of RA and is characterized by new blood vessel formation and the presence of infiltrative mononuclear cells such as macrophages and T lymphocytes.

Presentation

History

The characteristic history is waking in the middle of the night with pain and stiffness in the spine, in the cervical, dorsal or lumbar region. The patient may get out of bed and walk around to relieve the symptoms before returning to bed.

- On waking for the day, there is prolonged early morning stiffness that can last up to several hours. There is some improvement of symptoms during the day with worsening again in the evenings. This characteristic diurnal pattern is based on the fact that inflammation exacerbation is greater at night when cortisol levels are low.
- Associated problems include tenderness at various entheses where there is enthesopathy. Problems are characterized by pain and tenderness on palpation of points that may be widely distributed. Pain can be very distressing.

- There may be peripheral inflammatory arthritis but this is usually oligoarticular arthritis involving mainly large joints. Knees and hips are most likely to be involved.
- In a small proportion of patients, there may be uveitis with a complaint of blurring of vision and eye pain.

The diagnosis is often missed in women, leading to significantly delayed diagnosis. Some patients may present with already well-established ankylosing spondylitis.

Clinical examination

- In early cases of ankylosing spondylitis, findings will consist of loss of spinal mobility that it is reduced in all planes. This is distinct from other forms of back pain, e.g., cervical or lumbar spondylosis, where loss of movement may occur only in one plane, for example, flexion. Movements are painful.
- There may be tenderness at points of enthesopathy.
- There may also be peripheral oligoarticular synovitis.
- In more advanced cases, dorsal kyphosis (a lumbar spine that moves little if at all) is likely, and a similarly restricted movement of the cervical spine which may adopt a flexed position with associated problems of forward vision.

The differential diagnosis

There is very little difficulty in establishing the diagnosis in a classic case. The differential diagnosis resolves around the question of whether this is ankylosing spondylitis or an associated spondylitis in the context of an inflammatory bowel disease, particularly Crohn's disease, psoriasis or reactive arthritis. Occasionally, metastatic bone disease in the lumbar spine may lead to loss of all spinal movements. This can be distinguished by the lack of a diurnal pattern in the pain and associated systemic features. The acute-phase response cannot be used to distinguish between metastatic bone disease and ankylosing spondylitis because it will be raised in both conditions.

Investigations

In primary care:

- X-ray of the thoracolumbar junction and the sacroiliac joints is usually sufficient to establish the diagnosis. The characteristic features are erosive changes accompanied by syndesmophyte formation. In more advanced cases, X-rays show the characteristic bamboo spine. ESR or CRP elevation may be used to confirm inflammation.
- The HLA-B27 test should not be done. Back pain is common in the population and 8% of the normal population are HLA-B27

"The diagnosis may often be missed in women, leading to significantly delayed diagnosis"

" The HLA-B27 test should not be done "

101

positive. Hence, a proportion of patients with back pain not due to ankylosing spondylitis will be HLA-B27 positive.

Specialist investigations:

- Occasionally, despite the very clear diurnal pattern of symptoms and other associated features, plain radiography of the spine and the sacroiliac joints does not show characteristic changes. MRI scan of the sacroiliac joints is the best method to detect early sacroiliitis.

Management

Physiotherapy and posture

Patients should be instructed in maintaining spinal mobility using regular exercises. The National Ankylosing Spondylosis Society organizes group physiotherapy classes in various parts of the country and patients should be advised to join such a group. In addition, patients should be advised about posture, to maintain good spinal posture despite ankylosis. The mattress should be soft but firm and patients should sleep with only one pillow.

Drug therapy

> ❝Anti-TNF biologics will be approved for use in ankylosing spondylitis in the near future and PCTs should consider funding them before they are reviewed by NICE ❞

- Spinal pain and stiffness in ankylosing spondylitis: the mainstay is NSAIDs or Cox-2s. Phenylbutazone is no longer available.
- Peripheral arthritis: either with sulphasalazine or methotrexate as used to treat RA.
- Spinal symptoms: treatment is unsatisfactory. No drug has licensed approval for this indication. RCTs show that TNF blockade, with the anti-TNF biologics, is effective to treat spinal disease with benefit even to patients with advanced disease. Anti-TNF therapy also controls the symptoms of enthesopathy and peripheral synovitis. Anti-TNF biologics will be approved for use in ankylosing spondylitis in the near future and PCTs should consider funding them before they are reviewed by NICE.
- Uveitis: by an ophthalmologist.

Follow-up and prognosis

With current treatments, there is progressive loss of spinal mobility leading to spinal fusion in a significant proportion of patients. No prognostic tests help the physician to advise a patient whether they will have severe or mild disease. NSAIDs and Cox-2s do not appear to have any effect on the progress of spinal disease. Sulphasalazine and methotrexate, although effective for peripheral arthritis, are minimally effective for enthesopathy and have no impact on spinal disease itself. It is therefore important for patients to maintain spinal mobility and good spinal posture by means of regular exercises. Systemic complications, such as amyloidosis, are extremely rare.

Psoriatic arthritis

This is arthritis, with or without spondylitis, occurring in a person with psoriasis. The diagnosis can also be made if a first-degree relative has psoriasis, whether this is accompanied by arthritis or spondylitis or not.

❝Psoriatic arthritis, with or without spondylitis, occurring in a person with psoriasis❞

Aetiology and pathogenesis

The initiating cause is unknown. Inflammation in the joints, spine and skin may be driven by common mechanisms. Inflammatory mediators such as TNFα and IL-1 are present in the joints and skin lesions. The ability of TNFα inhibitors, such as the biologics, to effect rapid resolution and clearance of skin lesions and improve joint inflammation and symptoms of spondylitis point to a common underlying pathogenetic mechanism. The genetics are not fully understood. Psoriasis appears to be linked to HLA-C6 and spondylitis is linked to HLA-B27, but there is no convincing link between the peripheral arthritis and any genetic factor.

Presentation

Psoriatic arthritis encompasses the following entities:

- mono- and oligoarticular inflammatory arthritis, especially affecting the knee or hip,
- polyarticular disease resembling RA but RF negative,
- very rapidly destructive peripheral arthritis called arthritis mutilans,
- inflammatory spinal disease of the ankylosing spondylitis type.

RA can occur in patients with psoriasis, which is characterized by the presence of RF.

History and examination

The presentation of these various forms of peripheral arthritides, with or without accompanying spondylitis, makes diagnosis difficult. The whole picture can be put into its proper perspective if the psoriasis is detected in the patient or if a family history of psoriasis in first-degree relatives is obtained. Arthritis mutilans is rarely a presenting feature of psoriatic arthritis as it takes some period of time to develop fully. Both the peripheral arthritis and spondylitis are characterized by prolonged early morning stiffness and pain, nocturnal waking and reduced joint and spinal movement.

The joints are swollen and hot and painful on palpation; they may have an effusion. Measures of spinal movement, such as the

❝Both the peripheral arthritis and spondylitis are characterized by prolonged early morning stiffness and pain, nocturnal waking and reduced joint and spinal movement❞

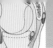

Schober index, and overall spinal movement are reduced during acute episodes of spondylitis or once spinal fusion has supervened after many years of disease activity. Occasionally, patients may present with uveitis. Patients should be warned that this complication can occur, what the symptoms are, and that they should seek emergency ophthalmological treatment.

Differential diagnosis

- Polyarticular psoriasis may be difficult to distinguish from RA unless RF is present.
- Mono- and oligoarticular arthritis cannot easily be distinguished from other such diseases in the absence of psoriasis or a history of psoriasis in the first-degree relatives.
- Just as psoriasis can occur years before arthritis, so it can occur years after the arthritis has first appeared.
- Where psoriasis is not present and there is no family history, ankylosing spondylitis, the arthritis of inflammatory bowel disease or even reactive arthritis should be considered.

Investigations

There are no specific diagnostic tests for psoriatic arthritis or psoriatic spondylitis. In primary care:

- RF may distinguish RA from polyarticular psoriatic arthritis.
- The acute-phase response is elevated.
- Plain radiographs may show erosive and destructive changes in some or all involved joints.
- Occasionally, serum uric acid may be elevated due to proliferation of skin cells. If one joint is more acutely inflamed and more painful than others, the possibility of gout should be considered. In this situation, elevated serum uric acid will suggest the diagnosis, which can be confirmed by examining joint fluid or tissue fluid under polarizing light for the presence of uric acid crystals.

The only specific investigations a rheumatologist may undertake is to aspirate joint or tissue fluid for microscopic examination.

Management

Drug management

- NSAIDs or Cox-2s may be used to control pain.
- Methotrexate is used for long-term management of both the psoriasis and arthritis, but this has no effect on the symptoms and signs of the spondylitic disease.
- Sulphasalazine has been used for the peripheral arthritis but with variable results. Antimalarials are contraindicated in the presence of psoriasis.

66 There are no specific diagnostic tests for psoriatic arthritis or psoriatic spondylitis 99

66 The possibility of gout should be considered 99

66 Methotrexate is used for long-term management of both the psoriasis and arthritis, but this has no effect on the symptoms and signs of the spondylitic disease 99

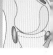

- Anti-TNF therapy will be the future drug treatment of choice for severe psoriatic arthropathy and psoriatic spondylitis. Current studies are exciting as there is currently no treatment that is effective in controlling the inflammation of spine. This treatment will be provided by a specialist rheumatology service.

❝ Anti-TNF therapy will be the future drug treatment of choice for severe psoriatic arthropathy and psoriatic spondylitis ❞

Physiotherapy and occupational therapy
Patients should be referred for physiotherapy and OT for specific problems. In patients with problems at home and in the work place, appropriate adjustments should be considered to improve access and function.

Diet
There is no evidence that diet plays any part in the management of psoriatic arthritis or spondylitis.

Follow-up and prognosis
- The outlook for patients with psoriatic arthritis and spondylitis has improved considerably over the last few years. In particular, peripheral arthritis can be managed very effectively with existing drug regimens.
- Mono- and oligoarticular forms of the disease generally have a very good prognosis.
- Polyarticular and arthritis mutilans disease are most likely to cause deformity, joint destruction, loss of function and consequent social isolation and loss of work.
- Anti-TNF therapy promises therapeutic success in the more intractable problem of the spondylitis.

Connective tissue diseases
Although the CTDs are rare, they should be considered in the differential diagnosis of a number of presenting manifestations. CTDs are also important because of the high morbidity and increased mortality with which they are associated. Primary SjS is the most common CTD, affecting 6–10 people/1000, while SLE is much rarer, affecting only 1/2000 of the UK population (Fig. 50).

Occurrence of connective tissue diseases
In a practice population of 2000 individuals:
• 12–20 patients will have Sjögren's syndrome
• 1 patient will have systemic lupus erythematosus
• 1–2 patients will have other connective tissue diseases

Fig. 50 Occurrence of connective tissue diseases

The CTDs are so called because of inflammation that, at one time, was thought to be confined to the connective tissues. The spectrum of disease that is now included under this label has vastly increased over the years and includes diseases that have a very targeted pathology, e.g., myositis, to more diffuse diseases such as SLE.

Aetiology and pathogenesis

The aetiology of the CTDs is unknown. Environmental agents may precipitate some CTDs, e.g., drug-induced SLE. The pathogenesis is thought to be dependent on autoimmunity and may involve autoanti-bodies that can directly attack tissues and organs, the deposition of immune complexes, activation of T-cells and macrophages with inflammatory and tissue-destructive properties, and disturbed immune regulation due to genetic factors.

Presentation

CTDs can present in a variety of ways, some of them extremely subtly, so the diagnosis may be delayed for some time. Presenting features may be divided into the non-specific (Fig. 51) and the specific

Fig. 51 Non-specific features of connective tissue disease presentation

Non-specific features of connective tissue disease presentation
• Arthralgia • Myalgia • Depression • Malaise • Weight loss • Fever • Lymphadenopathy

Fig. 52 Specific features of connective tissue diseases

Specific features of connective tissue diseases

• Raynaud's phenomenon
• Dryness of the occlusal surfaces
• Inflammatory arthritis in rashes:
   - Photosensitivity
   - Occlusal ulceration
   - Skin tightness/puffiness of digits
• Muscle weakness
• Recurrent unexplained fetal loss equal to or more than three usually in the mid trimester
• Pleurisy in the absence of infection
• Vascular events at an early age

(Fig. 52). The presence of one or more of the specific features in combination with non-specific features increases the likelihood of CTD.

Raynaud's phenomenon

Raynaud's phenomenon (RP) presents with the classic triphasic colour response: white digits during vascular spasm followed by blue digits due to partial spasm and impaired blood flow and, finally, red digits during the hyperaemic phase. It is important that this sequence of events is obtained during the history. RP occurs in about 5% of the general population. Primary RP usually begins in the teens and early twenties and is rarely associated with a CTD. The development of secondary RP in an older person may be a presentation of CTD. A careful search for non-specific and specific features of CTD as well as appropriate investigations should then be made. Features that may be present and suggest the presence of CTD are:

- year round symptoms with or without ulceration,
- abnormal nail fold capillaries viewed with an ophthalmoscope with a +20 lens,
- asymmetric upper limb pulses,
- tightness or puffiness of the fingers of the skin,
- elevated ESR,
- positive ANA,
- antibodies to ENA.

> *The classic triphasic colour response: white digits during vascular spasm followed by blue digits due to partial spasm and impaired blood flow and, finally, red digits during the hyperaemic phase*

Dryness of mucosal surfaces

The mucosal surfaces of the mouth, eyes, nose and vagina are commonly involved. Primary SjS may occur on its own without any other connective tissue or inflammatory joint disease. Secondary SjS may occur in the context of other CTDs and inflammatory joint diseases such as RA, SLE and systemic sclerosis. It is important to exclude other causes of dryness such as the menopause, diabetes mellitus and drugs such as antidepressants.

Features suggestive of SjS are shown in Fig. 53. The inflammatory arthritis is characterized by:

- early morning pain and stiffness lasting > 45 minutes,
- only minor evidence of soft-tissue swelling in most CTDs.

Patients with objective evidence of inflammatory arthritis should be referred for a specialist opinion, as this may also be the presenting manifestation of RA.

> *Secondary SjS may occur in the context of other CTDs and inflammatory joint diseases*

Skin rashes

A number of skin rashes are associated with CTDs:

- photosensitivity skin rashes, usually diffuse and erythematosus

Fig. 53 Features of
Sjögren's syndrome

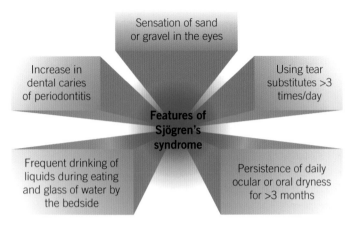

with or without blistering; on the face, it may be in the classic butterfly distribution,

- recurrent ulceration of the oral and nasal mucosa,
- discoid lupus, a discrete raised rash associated with hyperkeratosis, results in scarring and pigment changes,
- hair loss, frequently patchy, often permanent and may be associated with discoid lupus,
- in systemic sclerosis, skin tightening initially due to oedema of the skin and later due to fibrosis.

Muscle symptoms

Muscle symptoms are common. Subjective and objective muscle weakness may be accompanied by tenderness and wasting. In PMR, muscle weakness is due to pain and there is no objective evidence of muscle weakness.

Investigations

"A low positive ANA in the absence of clinically relevant symptoms and signs should not be taken to be evidence of a CTD"

Diagnosis of a CTD is difficult. A low positive ANA in the absence of clinically relevant symptoms and signs should not be taken as evidence of a CTD. The following investigations may help:

- Review the clinical notes to ascertain whether there has been an accumulation over time of relevant specific and non-specific features.
- Leukopenia (< 4 x 10^9/L), lymphopenia (< 1.5 x 10^9/L), thrombocytopenia (< 100 x 10^9/L) can be determined in primary care.
- Proteinuria and haematuria on dipstick examination of the urine is useful. Measurement of serum creatinine is useful but, by the time it is elevated, there is significant renal functional impairment.
- Creatine kinase is useful for diagnosis of polymyositis or dermatomyositis.

- ESR is frequently raised during exacerbation of CTDs but CRP may be normal in SLE when the ESR is elevated.
- Serological tests always cause problems. Screening tests should include ANA (to diagnose SLE) and ENA (to diagnose SjS and other CTDs including scleroderma and polymyositis). However, the interpretation of autoantibody tests may require advice from a rheumatologist.

66 The interpretation of autoantibody tests may require advice from a rheumatologist 99

The patient should be referred to a rheumatologist for:
- a high clinical index of suspicion,
- evolution of features suggestive of CTDs,
- positive screening serological (ANA and ENA) and other tests.

If in doubt and if there is evidence of major organ or tissue involvement, refer.

The rheumatologist will carry out further tests, including autoantibody and renal function tests. Patients with suspected SjS should preferably be referred to specialist, combined rheumatology/oral medicine departments where the problems of oral dental hygiene (caries, candida infection of the mouth and periodontitis) can be tackled effectively. They will undergo tests for pulmonary function and pulmonary hypertension, estimation of ENA antibodies, and measures of eye dryness (Schirmer's test) and parotid and total salivary flow. The investigation of patients with SLE may include CT scans and MRI scans. In women with suspected primary antiphospholipid syndrome, on the grounds of venous or arterial thrombosis or recurrent spontaneous abortions, a full workup of the clotting system is indicated.

Management

Acute problems in patients with CTDs are usually managed by the specialist. The GP has an integral role in the follow-up of such patients since these conditions are chronic and characterized by relapses and remissions. GPs can be particularly helpful in the following aspects of long-term care:
- monitoring and maintaining normal blood pressure,
- monitoring the toxicity and efficacy of immunosuppressive drugs,
- contraception, pregnancy and hormone replacement therapy in the context of the diagnosis,
- treating infection promptly, as it may trigger a flare of the disease,
- providing pneumococcal and annual influenza vaccinations as immunosuppressive therapy may exacerbate infections; beware of using statins, which can produce myositis in patients with polymyositis or dermatomyositis,
- monitoring for malignancy, because:
    - higher than normal risk of non-Hodgkin's lymphoma and maltome (lymphoma) in the salivary glands in SjS,

66 Providing pneumococcal and annual influenza vaccinations as immuno-suppressive therapy may exacerbate infections 99

– malignancy increases in association with dermatomyositis,

    – women on immunosuppressive therapy at increased risk of cervical disease; they should have regular cervical smears.

❝PMR and GCA are systemic inflammatory diseases of elderly people❞

Polymyalgia rheumatica/giant cell arteritis

PMR and GCA are systemic inflammatory diseases of people older than 50 years and are more common in people of northern European descent. Both conditions show a dramatic and favourable response to adequate doses of glucocorticoids.

GCA is a primary vasculitic disease. Other such diseases are rare: Takayasu's arteritis involves large arteries; polyarteritis nodosa and Kawasaki disease involve medium-sized arteries; Wegener's granulomatosis involves small arteries; and cryoglobulinaemia, cutaneous leucocytoclastic vasculitis and Henoch-Schönlein purpura involve arterioles/capillary venules.

Polymyalgia rheumatica

The features of PMR are summarized in Fig. 54. The pain and stiffness is worse in the mornings. There is a dramatic clinical response to glucocorticoids.

Aetiology and pathogenesis

The aetiology of PMR is unknown. The pathogenesis is also unclear as, apart from the acute-phase response, there are no biochemical or

Fig. 54 Features of polymyalgia rheumatica

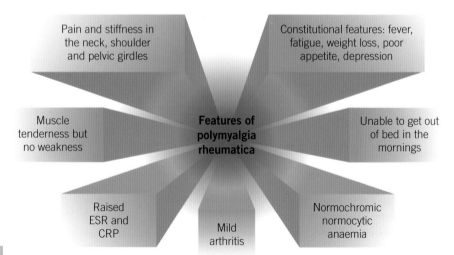

histological abnormalities. It may be a capsulitis of the shoulder and pelvic girdles. The occasional development of vasculitic occlusion such as in the retinal artery, histologically similar to that in GCA, suggests that there may be a vascular inflammatory component.

Presentation

History

The patient usually presents acutely with a complaint of waking up with stiffness and pain in the neck, shoulder and pelvic girdles with an inability to get out of bed. Sometimes the patient wakes during the night. Constitutional symptoms, such as malaise, fever and loss of weight, may occur. There may be mild arthritis and difficulty turning over in bed.

Examination

Despite the severity of the constitutional symptoms, clinical findings are sparse. The patient complains of tenderness in the muscles but muscle strength is normal within the limits of the pain. There may be mild synovitis of the wrists and the knees but polyarthritis does not occur.

Investigations

In primary care, patients usually present with a moderate to high ESR elevation, serum CRP elevation and normochromic normocytic anaemia. Despite marked muscle tenderness, muscle creatine kinase is normal. In secondary care, there are no specialist investigations, although biopsy of the temporal artery may be undertaken if there is a suspicion that the myalgic symptoms are part of GCA.

Management

The mainstay of management of PMR is prednisolone, starting at 15mg and reduced by 2.5mg every 6 weeks to 10mg daily and then by 1mg every 4 weeks. If the ESR becomes elevated or symptoms return, the previous dose of prednisolone should be given for a further 4 weeks before a further reduction is attempted. A maintenance dose of 5–7mg daily may be necessary for 6–12 months but there are no laboratory tests or other indicators to signal when the disease has "burnt itself out".

❝The mainstay of management of PMR is prednisolone❞

Follow-up and prognosis

In most patients, the disease persists for up to 5 years and unusually less than 2 years. There is no recognised steroid-sparing agent, although methotrexate has been given.

> *Most patients should receive prophylactic bone protective therapy*

> *GCA is a granulomatous vasculitis that commonly involves the arteries arising from the arch of the aorta*

Prophylaxis from steroid-induced osteoporosis
Most patients should receive prophylactic bone protective therapy, following the Royal College of Physicians guidelines (appendix 4).

Giant cell arteritis
GCA is a granulomatous vasculitis that commonly involves the arteries arising from the arch of the aorta.

Aetiology and pathogenesis
The aetiology of GCA is unknown. Histological examination of involved cranial arteries shows inflammatory changes with accumulation of mononuclear cells and formation of giant cells due to coalescence of macrophages. The internal elastic lamina of the artery is disrupted and there is excessive production of cytokines within the vasculitic lesion.

Presentation
Fig. 55 shows the features of GCA. Patients usually present acutely with:
- headaches, usually in the temporal region but occasionally in other regions of the scalp,
- systemic complaints such as weight loss, malaise, and fever.

Up to 30% of patients may also have symptoms characteristic of PMR.
- A minority of patients may present with:
  - claudication of the jaw muscles when eating,
  - occipital headaches due to involvement of the occipital arteries,
  - pain on combing their hair,
  - blurring of the vision or even frank sudden onset of blindness.

Fig. 55 Features of giant cell arteritis

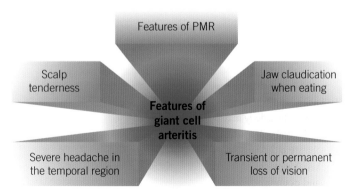

Features of PMR

Scalp tenderness

Jaw claudication when eating

Features of giant cell arteritis

Severe headache in the temporal region

Transient or permanent loss of vision

Examination

A clinical examination will demonstrate tenderness on palpation of the involved cranial artery. The temporal artery is enlarged and tortuous, with overlying inflamed skin, and tender on palpation. It does not pulsate. In patients with visual problems, fundoscopic examination may show optic nerve atrophy.

Investigations

In primary care, ESR and CRP are both abnormally elevated. Patients should be referred to secondary care for a temporal artery biopsy, which may be negative in up to one-third or one-half of patients because of the localized nature of the lesions. Imaging is not usually indicated.

Management

Glucocorticoids are the mainstay of treatment. The starting dose of prednisolone is higher than for PMR usually being 30mg daily initially for 2 to 3 months reduced by 5mg every 4 weeks until the dose is 10mg daily. Thereafter the schedule is the same as for PMR. A somewhat higher dose of prednisolone (up to 60mg daily) is recommended for patients with ocular involvement but once visual loss has occurred, it is unlikely to return.

> ❝ *Glucocorticoids are the mainstay of treatment* ❞

Follow-up and prognosis

ESR is used to follow the disease and monitor treatment. The prognosis is good although complete resolution of the disease may take up to 5 years. It is important that glucocorticoid reduction is managed cautiously and effectively to prevent serious complications such as visual loss. No effective steroid-sparing agent has been described although methotrexate has been used.

Prophylaxis from steroid-induced osteoporosis

All patients should receive osteoporosis-preventing therapy as soon as glucocorticoids have been introduced, following the recommendations of the Royal College of Physicians of England (appendix 4).

> ❝ *All patients should receive osteoporosis-preventing therapy as soon as glucocorticoids have been introduced* ❞

Differential diagnosis of PMR/GCA

The differential diagnosis for PMR/GCA is fairly large (Fig. 56). In practice, a few simple screening tests are sufficient to exclude most of them.

- RA in the elderly may present as PMR. A careful clinical examination will reveal polyarthritis. Be suspicious if the patient is unable to reduce the steroid dosage or needs an increasing dosage (Case study 1).
- GCA may present as PMR. A careful history, clinical examination and examination of the cranial arteries, particularly the temporal

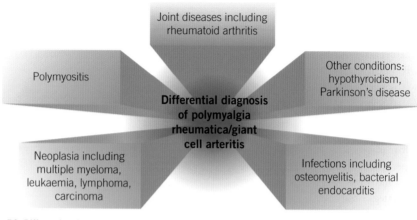

Fig. 56 **Differential diagnosis of polymyalgia rheumatica/giant cell arteritis**

arteries, will reveal symptoms, such as blurring of vision, that exclude this possibility.

- Malignancy may present with these features. A serum immunoglobulin concentration and electrophoresis will exclude multiple myeloma. Further investigations to exclude other malignant conditions should only be carried out if indicated.
- The most likely muscle disease is polymyositis, which can be excluded by the fact that there is no muscle weakness in PMR and the serum creatine kinase is normal.

Patient education and self-management programmes

Patient education

66 Today's delivery of care is all about improving patients' knowledge, confidence and coping abilities in relation to their problems 99

Today's delivery of care is all about improving patients' knowledge, confidence and coping abilities in relation to their problems. This means providing education, information and support. Written information needs to be explained or used to reinforce information given during a one-to-one or group session. Patients respond to different strategies and materials, which may include:

- patient leaflets/written information, such as those provided by **arc** and Arthritis Care (appendix 6),
- audio or video tapes,
- use of allied health professionals,
- telephone contact,
- group education/activities,

- individual management plans developed after the use of question cue and response interview (self-management programmes),
- interactive computer programmes,
- internet and intranet information and self-help programmes, e.g., MOVE website exercise programme,
- self-help groups such as those organised by Arthritis Care, Ankylosing Spondylitis and Pain Society,
- patient support organisations, e.g., Arthritis Care, NRAS (appendix 6),
- self-management programmes,
- expert patient programmes, e.g., Department of Health/Arthritis Care Initiatives.

These strategies and materials need to be individually focused. Patient needs will change depending upon the stage of the illness, age, personality and social interaction (Fig. 57).

Self-management programmes

Approximately 25% of people with a specific condition seek medical advice. Musculoskeletal consultations accounted for 19.5% of all GP appointments in 1991–92, an increase of 4.3% over 1981–82, which was an increase of 46% over the figures for 1971–72. It is difficult to know why the demand has increased. It may be due to increasing affluence, higher expectations and the fact that people live longer. A small increase at this level produces a major increase in workload even if the referral rate to secondary care does not change.

These increases have produced major changes in the delivery of care and management, with more reliance on practice nurses, community physiotherapists and the recent formal development of GPs with a special interest (GPwSI), who often work within a multidisciplinary team with links to orthopaedics, rheumatology and plastic surgery.

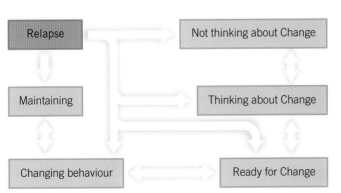

Fig. 57 Ready for change. Reprinted from Chronic Condition Self-Management Guidelines – Summary for Nurses and Allied Health Professionals, RACGP.

115

From the patient perspective, there are now many things on offer. Most people have access to exercise programmes, but the most exciting developments are the self-management programmes for chronic diseases developed initially in the USA but greatly extended by the UK, Canada and Australia. Australia has produced material to help evaluate and decide which patients are ready for change, using a question cue and response interview (appendix 4) designed to suggest questions to define how the patient understands his/her disease or condition, whether or not more education and understanding is necessary, and what other help may be required. In the USA, a self-help course has been shown to reduce pain by 20% and physician visits by 40%. Health education for self-management in patients with chronic arthritis has sustained health benefits while reducing health care costs.

The Department of Health (DOH) is working with various organisations and personnel developing "the expert patient", another self-management initiative. All rely on a mixture of personnel and educational material. **arc** and Arthritis Care have produced many booklets and web-based resources and the DOH has produced booklets for their expert patient courses that can be purchased on similar lines to the *Back Book*.

Do these programmes work?

The benefits to patients appear to be modest but they do produce reductions in pain, fatigue and health distress with increases in physical activity and self-efficacy. These changes are equivalent to the benefits achieved by many pharmacological agents but the programmes can be delivered to a large number of people at relatively low cost. This should mean that the societal benefits are substantial.

Physical therapy

The role of the physiotherapist in musculoskeletal medicine (MSK) is fast expanding and seems to be limited only by the availability of trained personnel. Community physiotherapists are nearly all senior therapists who have a wealth of experience. Most PCTs have increased the number of physiotherapists and have encouraged GPs to refer patients directly to them in order to ease the pressure on orthopaedic referrals. Physiotherapists should be the cornerstone of the new multidisciplinary teams managing MSK. They are excellent in assessing and managing MSK problems and have the communication skills needed to explain and teach self-management exercise programmes and complement the GP skills of diagnosis and individual patient management. This resource must not be abused by inappropriate referrals, e.g., patients with knee OA who are unlikely to comply with exercise regimes.

66 Physiotherapists are excellent in assessing and managing MSK problems and have the communication skills needed to explain and teach self-management exercise programmes and complement the GP skills of diagnosis and individual patient management 99

Modalities used by physiotherapists

Physiotherapy has moved away from using static machines as there is little evidence to support their use. Current regimes include:

- stretching,
- balance/co-ordination,
- relaxation,
- manipulation,
- hydrotherapy,
- ice/heat,
- gait analysis,
- TENS,
- acupuncture,
- ultrasound,
- injections,
- orthotics,
- patella taping.

Appointments with physiotherapists are longer than those with GPs and are used to give quality help and information to the patient and referring physician. Patients are given a full assessment, excellent education and usually a self-management regime. Follow-up appointments and additional treatment modalities are given where appropriate.

Hydrotherapy

- Water is an ideal environment for exercise because it makes the body "weightless". Many community pools have exercise sessions with a physiotherapist in attendance. This may be a way to encourage patients with OA of the large joints to increase their activities.
- Hydrotherapy has always been of value to patients with flares of RA or ankylosing spondylitis.
- Research projects are underway to assess the benefits of hydrotherapy.

66 Water is an ideal environment for exercise because it makes the body "weightless" 99

Ice/heat

It is not possible to predict when heat or ice may help arthritic joints. Cold is more likely to relieve painful joints that have been overused or are inflamed.

Ice (cryotherapy) is incorporated into the early stages of management of soft tissue injuries in sport using the RICE principle:

- rest,
- ice,
- compression,
- elevation.

Cold is often good for relieving pain following injury or surgery. Apply an ice pack (a bag of frozen peas is ideal) wrapped in a towel to the

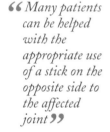

affected area for not more than 20 minutes. Heat may also ease pain. The home remedy is a bean bag that is heated in the microwave.

Gait analysis and joint protection

Analysis and re-education is a priority for patients with inflammatory arthritis where maintaining quality of life and independence is vital. Physiotherapists and occupational therapists will give advice on joint protection and aids for the home. Request advice and help for patients with OA. The use of neat, comfortable and easy-to-wear CMC supports is especially helpful for thumb OA, especially when pursuing particular activities (appendix 5).

Many patients can be helped with the appropriate use of a stick on the opposite side to the affected joint. The stick should come up to the crease at the wrist. To check this, with the patient standing straight, turn the stick upside down and mark the level of the wrist crease on the stick; cut the stick to this length, then attach a ferule. Check the ferule for wear occasionally and replace it if necessary.

Podiatrists (or an orthotist) may work with a physiotherapist to assess foot and lower limb problems. In future, these clinics may include a podiatric surgeon; some PCTs already have these combined clinics. Communicating these important changes to all members of the primary care team will ensure their success. These teams may also give advice about childhood gait problems.

66 Many patients can be helped with the appropriate use of a stick on the opposite side to the affected joint 99

**Fig 58 Spenco®
Polysorb Cross Trainer
replacement insole.**
Reprinted with
permission from Spenco
Medical Corporation.

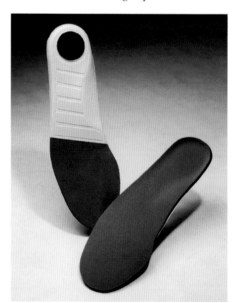

Shoes

Shock-absorbing footwear is considered beneficial for anyone with joint pains. Trainers are ideal but if these are unacceptable to the patient, commercial alternatives are Ecco, Hotter or Padders. Other compromises are discussed under insoles.

Insoles/orthotics

Patients with major gait problems, especially those with inflammatory arthritis, require specialist podiatry advice. Most patients who have lower limb OA or tendonitis may be helped using an off-the-shelf appliance for common, straightforward problems. More complicated cases must be referred for gait analysis or full podiatry assessment.

Crosstrainer replacement sorbothane insoles (with arch support and heel pad)

These insoles (Fig. 58) are used for:

- Plantar fasciitis.
- Hypermobile patients with knee pain. Useful in making walking and athletic activities less painful. In essence, they convert ordinary shoes into trainers.
- Patients with hip OA, knee and trochanteric bursitis. The mechanics are altered, changing the forces through the body and hopefully the amount of pain. Put insoles into steel-capped work boots and Wellingtons to reduce discomfort and pain.
- Bruised heel syndrome and some patients with Achilles tendon problems; excellent results are achieved.

Thin sorbothane Insoles

Primary care is about achieving the possible and for patients who only wear court shoes and cannot be persuaded to wear lace-ups or shock absorbing shoes these insoles are a useful compromise.

> **" Primary care is about achieving the possible "**

³/₄ arch sorbothane cushion insoles (not rigid)

These are used for:

- Achilles tendonitis, classically seen in overweight females who only wear slip-on shoes. The ³/₄ arch supports correct all the mechanics (flat feet and stressed lateral border of the Achilles tendon) and give pain relief (Fig. 59).
- Patients with OA of large joints who wear only slip-on shoes or sandals. The ³/₄ insoles allow this type of footwear to be worn.

Fig. 59 Large woman and fridge. Overweight patients have: pronated flat feet, a tendency to wear only slip-on shoes, anserine bursitis, Achilles tendonitis (pain on the lateral border of the tendon) and pain in the mid foot. Reprinted from The Sunday Times Business Section, 6th July 2003, with permission from Masterfile.

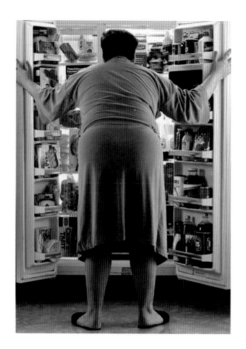

4° (¹/₄ inch) heel wedge

These may be tried to change the mechanics and so prevent/reduce medial knee pain in OA. The high side of the wedge is placed on the lateral side of the shoes so that this side is higher and the weight is taken here rather than at the medial side (the medial tibiofemoral compartment is usually primarily and more severely affected in knee OA). These wedges are inexpensive and may give as much relief as analgesics. Heel wedges may also be used to correct heel varus and valgus but podiatry referral is usually advised.

Metatarsal domes

These are useful for patients complaining of metatarsalgia, but podiatric advice should also be sought.

Cushions/raises

Some patients have a degree of leg-length discrepancy following a hip or knee arthroplasty and will walk with a limp and may develop trochanteric bursitis. Quite often, these patients will benefit from a sorbothane heel insert in the shoe of the shorter leg. This is a practical solution that is always worth trying as rarely is the leg-length discrepancy enough to warrant full podiatric gait assessment.

Double-strap Vulkan support for tennis/golfers elbow
The support gives the patient confidence to use the elbow again and to return to, or continue at, work. It is easy to use and is unlikely to be applied incorrectly, i.e., over the painful enthesitis (Fig. 28, page 57). The important principle is not to use too large a support.

Wrist supports for carpal tunnel syndrome
These supports will relieve symptoms in 80% of patients. They should be fitted so that the wrist is held in the neutral position.

Exercise
Stretching exercises
These are important for many muscle and tendon problems. During healing, some contraction takes place, so ligaments and tendons become minimally shorter and therefore more prone to further or chronic injury. A good example of this is a sprained ankle. Patients with tennis/golfers enthesopathies should also stretch the relevant tendons, especially on waking and regularly during the day.

Quadriceps exercises and exercise regimes
- All patients with joint pains will benefit from exercises to develop muscles to protect the relevant joint(s). Developing quadriceps muscles for knee pain is the classic example.
- Usually, this is a specific programme of isometric, isotonic and resistive exercises. It is important to demonstrate these exercises to the patient to improve compliance and confidence. The **arc** knee OA patient leaflet gives two good examples and the MOVE website contains an evidence-based exercise programme for patients with knee OA: further programmes will be added.
- Patients should be encouraged to continue, or to take up new, hobbies and leisure pursuits that will improve their physical fitness. This is particularly important for patients with hypermobility who have more joint pain and stiffness when activities are restricted.
- The National Ankylosing Spondylitis support groups organise group exercise sessions, usually in a gymnasium but some groups have access to hydrotherapy/swimming pools. Primary care must encourage patients to join these support groups.

Exercise prescriptions
The change in emphasis and delivery of health care towards primary care has encouraged community-based projects to promote better health. There are different ways to access these projects but patients are usually referred for exercise sessions by a health professional and

❝All patients with joint pains will benefit from exercises to develop muscles to protect the relevant joint(s)❞

❝Patients should be encouraged to continue, or to take up new, hobbies and leisure pursuits that will improve their physical fitness. This is particularly important for patients with hypermobility who have more joint pain and stiffness when activities are restricted❞

Fig. 60 Poster for self-referral programme

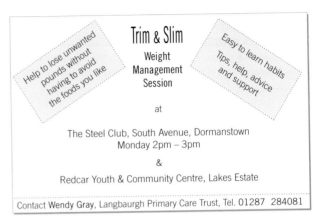

Trim & Slim

Weight Management Session

Help to lose unwanted pounds without having to avoid the foods you like

Easy to learn habits Tips, help, advice and support

at

The Steel Club, South Avenue, Dormanstown
Monday 2pm – 3pm

&

Redcar Youth & Community Centre, Lakes Estate

Contact Wendy Gray, Langbaurgh Primary Care Trust, Tel. 01287 284081

self-refer for others (Fig. 60). Many similar schemes are run in health or community localities.

Exercise by Prescription

Exercise by Prescription, run by Langbaurgh PCT, is an example of the type of scheme that can be used to prescribe exercise. It is a 10–15-week course of exercise sessions led by qualified instructors. Each session lasts 1–2 hours and clients are welcome to attend 1–3 sessions/week. Sessions are suitable for people suffering from a wide range of health problems. Exercise can have a profound effect on health and well-being, offering both physical and mental health benefits in a preventative and rehabilitative way.

> **"Those who are physically inactive often find taking the first step into exercise is the most difficult "**

Those who are physically inactive often find taking the first step into exercise is the most difficult. On the *Exercise by Prescription* scheme, different activities and individual exercise programmes allow people with varying degrees of mobility and fitness to exercise within their capabilities alongside other referrals of similar abilities. Activities include:

- gym-based exercise (supervised),
- gentle exercise classes,
- swimming/water-based exercise,
- health issue discussions,
- light circuit training.

Clients on the scheme are by referral only. GPs, practice nurses, physiotherapists or other medical professional can refer a client. Venues include adult education centres, leisure centres, sports academies and a Civic Hall. There is a small charge for the use of facilities, which varies from venue to venue. Clients who need assistance showering or changing can bring a friend or carer. There is a follow-up class to the scheme called *Step Ahead*. This class is ongoing and is used to maintain and promote fitness and mobility levels.

Other modalities

TENS and acupuncture

These modalities are useful adjuncts to other treatments, especially for patients with chronic pain, e.g., back, neck and shoulder pain, poly-arthralgia and fibromyalgia.

Alternative physical treatments

Treatments such as reflexology, yoga classes, Tai Chi, relaxation classes, manipulation techniques and Pilates may help in patient management.

Ultrasound and shock absorption

Ultrasound is used to treat areas of musculoskeletal inflammation such as enthesitis, trochanteric bursitis, plantar fasciitis and Achilles tendonitis. These common conditions are usually seen in isolation but may be part of a more generalized condition such as ankylosing spondylitis.

Shock absorption therapy uses sound waves generated in water by an electro-hydraulic or electromagnetic source. There is growing interest in this type of therapy for enthesopathies, for example plantar fasciitis, and the results from good prospective studies are awaited with interest.

Patella taping

This is a simple but rarely used technique. Investigated in 1994 and 2003, it seems to be most useful in relieving patellofemoral pain (anterior knee pain). It is usually the lateral half of the patella that is affected (compare medial compartment for tibiofemoral OA). Taping is assumed to correct patella malalignment, reducing pain during walking and climbing stairs.

- Shave the skin prior to tape application.
- Apply hypoallergenic under-tape (e.g., Fixomull) beneath the rigid tape to prevent irritation.
- Apply two pieces of rigid tape (e.g., Leuko Sports tape premium plus) with the patella pushed medially and correct any lateral and anteroposterior tilt.
- Apply two pieces of rigid tape below the patella over the infra-patellar fat pad.

Occupational therapy

Aids and appliances enable patients to function better and be as independent as possible. Hobbies must not be forgotten when assessing patients. Many simple aids are greatly appreciated, e.g., a rack for holding playing cards or a book.

> *Treatments such as reflexology, yoga classes, Tai Chi, relaxation classes, manipulation techniques and Pilates may help in patient management*

> *Aids and appliances enable patients to function better and be as independent as possible. Hobbies must not be forgotten when assessing patients*

123

" Any treatment given to a patient should be appropriate for the individual and their disease. Use the least potentially dangerous drugs as first choice, i.e., analgesics (simple or compound), to give pain relief that is acceptable to the patient "

" The important principle is to strive to give the patient maximum pain relief and mobility in the safest possible way while respecting the patient's views and opinions "

Pharmacological therapy

Management priorities and strategies vary with each disease/condition and with the individual. Drugs are an important part of management for:

- symptom control (analgesics, NSAIDs, Cox-2s),
- prevention of long-term damage (DMARDs),
- decreasing or modifying inflammation (steroids, NSAIDS, Cox-2s).

Many patients in primary care have a healthy scepticism about taking tablets and are often only willing to try tablets or steroid injections as a last resort. These patients can often be helped by appropriate physical therapy, with or without topical treatments, or the occasional analgesic. Unfortunately, a few will require a full pharmacological armamentarium, e.g., patients with RA. In these instances, the skills of both the primary and secondary care team will be needed to achieve patient compliance and disease control. This scenario is seen in chronic diseases of all systems.

Practical considerations for osteoarthritis and musculoskeletal problems

Any treatment given to a patient should be appropriate for the individual and their disease. Use the least potentially dangerous drugs as first choice, i.e., analgesics (simple or compound), to give pain relief that is acceptable to the patient. Most patients can be managed this way, sometimes with the addition of topical treatments. Some patients will require either the addition, or the replacement, of the analgesic with NSAIDs/Cox-2s. UK practitioners should use NICE guidance for this. The important principle is to strive to give the patient maximum pain relief and mobility in the safest possible way while respecting the patient's views and opinions.

Topical agents
Rubefacients

There is no evidence to support their use but they are inexpensive, have few side effects and have been used for many years. They are usually bought over the counter (OTC preparations).

Topical NSAIDs

There is some evidence to support the use of topical NSAIDs in chronic pain conditions such as OA. They are significantly better than placebo over a 2-week period, with a number needed to treat (NNT) of 3.1 (appendix 5).

- Topical therapy greatly reduces the risk of developing serious side effects compared with other drug treatments. If a patient finds this beneficial, it is often cost effective as the patient may not require analgesics or oral NSAIDs or drugs to treat side effects.

- There is doubt about the exact mechanism of action of topical NSAIDs. Is the act of rubbing or massage effective? Drug levels within the joint indicate direct absorption through the skin, which may account for the efficacy.
- Most are available OTC as well as on prescription. As with oral preparations, patients should be advised to try more than one type.

Capsaicin

Capsaicin is derived from hot chillies. It probably acts by entering the joint and depleting substance P, a neuropeptide involved in the transmission of pain in the afferent fibres. It is safe, but on application, produces burning or tingling sensations in approximately 50% of patients. This usually settles within a few weeks but it is sensible to wash the hands after applying the cream, to avoid contact with sensitive parts of the body such as the eyes. Capsaicin is available on prescription only in Europe and the USA.

Both the ACR and the Primary Care Rheumatology Society, in their respective guidelines for OA management, suggest capsaicin be tried after paracetamol and before oral NSAIDs/Cox-2s (appendix 4).

Which topical treatments can be used as an adjunct to oral therapy?

- All three treatments can be used in conjunction with analgesics.
- Only rubefacients and capsaicin can be prescribed with oral NSAIDs/Cox-2s.
- Sometimes topical NSAIDs and paracetamol are the only relatively safe treatments for patients with severe cardiovascular problems or severe, present or past, gastrointestinal problems. This latter group may include patients with Crohn's disease, who often have exacerbation of their Crohn's if they take oral NSAIDs/Cox-2s.
- Patients who develop hypertension or renal problems when taking oral NSAIDs/Cox-2s may also benefit from topical treatment.

Patient misconceptions concerning medications and responses

"Pain killers merely mask the symptoms and do not treat the underlying condition"

It is important to counsel patients so that they understand that analgesics are the correct treatment for many conditions and that often NSAIDs/Cox-2s are not appropriate. The aim is to give enough pain relief to maintain or retain mobility, so maintaining muscle strength.

❝ Sometimes topical NSAIDs and paracetamol are the only relatively safe treatments for patients with severe cardiovascular problems or severe, present or past, gastrointestinal problems ❞

125

"I can buy it over the counter so it cannot be very effective"
This perception may be the reason for the statement, "I want some stronger painkillers, doctor". Often it transpires that the patient's self-help regime is inadequate and an explanation of how to take paracetamol, with or without codeine, is time well spent.

Fear of addiction

This fear is seen most often in patients who take paracetamol 8/day (4g daily) for pain relief. There is no evidence that paracetamol alone is addictive though, if combined with an opiate, some patients become dependent. This does not happen often in patients with chronic conditions such as RA or OA. Caution: The *BNF* (British National Formulary) lists that prolonged/regular use of paracetamol may enhance the effects of warfarin.

Simple and compound analgesics/opioids

Analgesics, simple and compound, are the mainstay of musculoskeletal drug therapy. Their main use is to relieve pain in order to maintain function and activities. This is the same for acute and chronic conditions. They include:

- paracetamol, alone, with codeine, dihydrocodeine, or dextropropoxyphene,
- nefopam,
- meptazinol,
- tramadol.

Patients may require considerable encouragement and education to take these drugs appropriately.

Paracetamol

Paracetamol is a useful and effective drug that should be the first choice for pain relief.

- Patients need encouragement to take paracetamol in adequate doses and at regular intervals.
- It is safe for all ages if taken according to the manufacturer's instructions. It is associated with a negligible risk of gastrointestinal bleeding (1:1200 with NSAIDs) and has no cardiac toxicity; it is safe for patients with cardiac disease.
- Paracetamol is only dangerous in overdose. The maximum dose is 8 tablets (4g) daily.
- It does not cause:
  - perforations, ulcers or bleeds,
  - asthma; it is safe for asthmatics to use,

> *Analgesics, simple and compound, are the mainstay of musculoskeletal drug therapy. Their main use is to relieve pain in order to maintain function and activities. This is the same for acute and chronic conditions*

- Paracetamol can be added to adequate doses of codeine to give excellent NNTs: co-codamol 500mg + 8mg or 500mg + 30mg.
- It can be used as an adjunct to NSAIDs/Cox-2s.

Opiate drugs and newer alternatives

The opiate based drugs codeine, dihydrocodeine and dextropropoxyphene may cause constipation and drowsiness and sometimes addiction.

The new analgesics may be useful in some patients but they all have side effects and their NNTs explain why they are not first choices.

Nefopam hydrochloride

A non-narcotic, benzoxazine analgesic useful for elderly patients with musculoskeletal conditions. It may give sympathetic and antimuscarinic side effects such as nervousness, headache, anxiety, vertigo, nausea, vomiting, blurred vision, sweating, insomnia, tachycardia and dysuria. The dose for the elderly is 30mg three times daily (range, 30–90mg tid). Patients need to be warned that it may turn urine pink.

Tramadol

This is an opiate analogue that, in theory, causes fewer opioid side effects. It also enhances serotoninergic and adrenergic pathways that may lead to side effects such as hypertension or hypotension, hallucinations and confusion as well as the usual morphine side effects of nausea, vomiting, constipation and drowsiness. It has an NNT of 5 so is rarely a first-line drug. If the patient tolerates tramadol, it is often an effective analgesic. It can be useful for patients with fibromyalgia.

Fentanyl

Apart from being given by injection for intra-operative analgesia, fentayl is available as a self-adhesive patch to be changed every 3 days. At present, there are only 25µg/hour, or greater, patches that are often too strong for elderly patients with moderate to severe OA.

Alternative opioid analgesics include:

- meptazinol,
- nalbuphine,
- pentazocine,
- buprenorphine,
- morphine,
- pethidine.

NSAIDs

NSAIDs are commonly prescribed for most musculoskeletal problems. Their main advantage over analgesics is that fewer daily doses are

"NSAIDs are commonly prescribed for most musculoskeletal problems"

Gastrointestinal	Renal	Central nervous system	Hypersensitivity	Cardiovascular
Peptic ulceration	Renal failure	Tinnitus	Rash	Fluid retention leading to heart failure and loss of hypertension control
Perforation of ulcer	Interstitial fibrosis	Photosensitivity	Bronchospasm	
Bleeding from peptic ulcer	Papillary necrosis	Headaches	Angio-oedema	
Dyspepsia	Bladder problems/ cystitis (tiaprofenic acid)	Personality changes		
Nausea				
Diarrhoea				
Iron deficiency anaemia from chronic gastrointestinal bleeding				
Colitis				

Fig. 61 NSAID side effects

required. They also relieve the stiffness of OA and RA. NSAIDs do not treat the arthritis but they do give pain relief and so increase mobility and the associated quality of life. NSAIDs also decrease inflammation and inflammatory swelling so they are excellent for treating gout. They share a major role with DMARDs in the treatment of RA. There is an inflammatory component to OA, which may be a major component in some patients, who usually respond well to NSAIDs and take them long-term.

Side effects

The disadvantage of NSAIDS is their side effects (Fig. 61), especially the hidden ones of sudden catastrophic bleeding from the gastrointestinal tract and interactions causing fluid retention and loss of blood pressure control in patients taking antihypertensive medications. It is estimated that 2300 people die each year in the UK from NSAID-

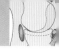

induced peptic ulcer, gastrointestinal perforations or bleeds. Often there is no warning of catastrophe, hence the term "hidden side effect". These problems led to the development of Cox-2s (Fig. 62).

Reducing gastrointestinal complications

The addition of misoprostol reduces gastrointestinal complications by 50%, reducing rather than eliminating the risks. Misoprostol also adds its own side effects (diarrhoea can be profound) and can produce all the gastrointestinal side effects caused by NSAIDs, including:

- nausea,
- vomiting,
- abdominal pain,
- dyspepsia,
- flatulence,
- vaginal bleeding.

Omeprazole and other proton pump inhibitors will reduce peptic ulceration and, presumably, ulcer complications, although there is no evidence for this. Simple measures to reduce gastrointestinal complications are:

- Use smallest dose of drug possible, especially in the elderly.
- Do not use two NSAIDs together.
- In the elderly, use topical treatments and simple/compound analgesics before NSAIDs.
- Take a good history about previous gastrointestinal problems, smoking and alcohol intake. NSAIDs are not recommended for heavy smokers and heavy drinkers.
- Use drugs that are less acidic in the stomach, e.g., nabumetone, or partially Cox-2 selective, e.g., meloxicam, etodolac.
- Use Cox-2s.

Fig. 62 Adverse events and gastrointestinal tolerability of clecoxib versus NSAIDs.
Reprinted from McKenna F, et al. *Clin Exp Rheumatol* 2002;20:35-43.

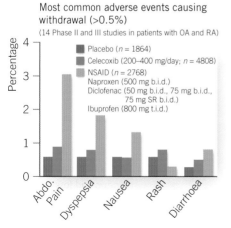

Most common adverse events causing withdrawal (>0.5%)
(14 Phase II and III studies in patients with OA and RA)

Placebo (n = 1864)
Celecoxib (200–400 mg/day; n = 4808)
NSAID (n = 2768)
Naproxen (500 mg b.i.d.)
Diclofenac (50 mg b.i.d., 75 mg b.i.d., 75 mg SR b.i.d.)
Ibuprofen (800 mg t.i.d.)

Percentage

Abdo. Pain · Dyspepsia · Nausea · Rash · Diarrhoea

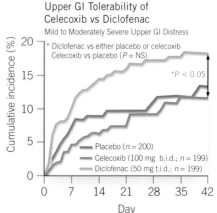

Upper GI Tolerability of Celecoxib vs Diclofenac
Mild to Moderately Severe Upper GI Distress

* Diclofenac vs either placebo or celecoxib
Celecoxib vs placebo (P = NS)

*$P < 0.05$

Cumulative incidence (%)

Placebo (n = 200)
Celecoxib (100 mg b.i.d.; n = 199)
Diclofenac (50 mg t.i.d.; n = 199)

Day

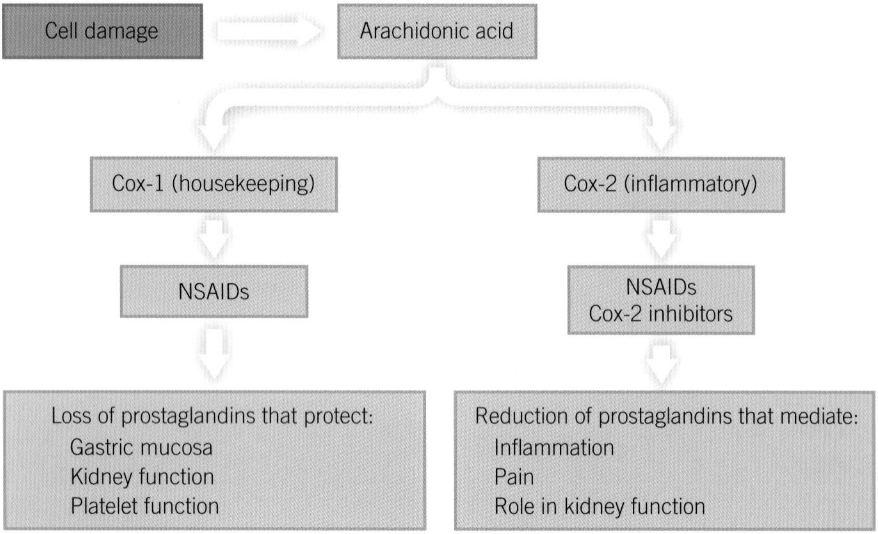

Fig. 63 Inhibition by classic NSAIDs and selective Cox-2 inhibitors

Lowest risk	Intermediate risk	High risk
Ibuprofen	Diclofenac	Azapropazone
	Indomethacin	
	Naproxen	
	Ketaprofen	
	Piroxicam	

Ibuprofen is probably only a low risk at low doses; at 2.4g/day, it will have the equivalent risk of the intermediate group. Even at this dosage, it is less expensive to prescribe and is presently the only oral NSAID available over the counter. Piroxicam comes at the high end of the intermediate group. Azapropazone should no longer be used as a routine NSAID.

Fig. 64 NSAID risk groups

How do NSAIDs work?

Sir John Vane suggested that this class of drug worked by inhibiting the synthesis of the prostaglandins that are essential for the development of inflammation. NSAIDs inhibit the enzyme cyclo-oxygenase that leads to the formation of inflammatory prostaglandins. There are two isoforms of cyclo-oxygenase.

Cox-1

This is the housekeeping constitutive cyclo-oxygenase enzyme involved in the production of several important products from arachidonic acid (Fig. 63):

- prostacyclin: protects the gastric mucosa,
- prostaglandin E_2: protects kidney function,
- thromboxane A_2: protects platelet function.

Cox-2

This inflammation-induced enzyme gives rise to the production from arachidonic acid of proteases, prostaglandins and inflammatory mediators involved in the inflammatory process (Fig. 63). Cox-2 also has a housekeeping role in maintaining kidney and other physiological functions.

Classic NSAIDs inhibit both Cox-1 and Cox-2 to varying degrees according to the specific generic compound. The Committee on the Safety of Medicines (CSM) reported the relative safety of NSAIDs in common use in 1994 (Fig. 64).

NICE has given Cox-2s the name coxibs. The second review of these drugs is underway. Cox-2s available/licensed to date include:

- refecoxib,
- celecoxib,
- etoricoxib,
- valdecoxib,
- lumiracoxib.

Etodolac and meloxicam are partially selective Cox-2s. Appendix 1 gives dosage and other details for all these drugs. A fifth Cox-2 specific inhibitor 'lumiracoxib' is currently in development. Full details of the drug are not yet available, however an 18,000 patient outcomes study 'TARGET' is expected to report in 2004 and will be the largest safety outcomes study yet conducted within this drug class.

Cox-2s reduce the number of serious gastrointestinal side effects, i.e., perforations, ulcers and bleeds (Fig. 65). Unfortunately, their overall risk-to-benefit ratio may depend on non-gastrointestinal events and this data is still controversial. Results from ongoing studies are eagerly awaited; only then can rational discussion be made about their use. NICE has produced useful guidance on their use in high-risk patients.

NICE guidance on Cox-2s

Cox-2s should be prescribed in preference to standard NSAIDs in patients considered to be at high risk of gastrointestinal complications. These include:

- patients > 65 years,
- patients with a history of peptic ulcer/gastrointestinal bleed/

Cox–2s should be prescribed in preference to standard NSAIDs in patients considered to be at high risk of gastrointestinal complications

131

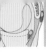

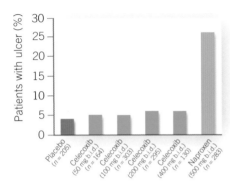

Celecoxib

Incidence of gastroduodenal ulcers – week 12
(Phase III RA and OA UGI safety trials)

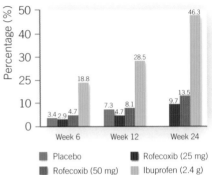

Rofecoxib

Cumulative gastric/duodenal ulcer incidence (≥3 mm)

* Significantly different from all other treatments;
  $P < 0.001$

Fig. 65 Incidence of ulcers using coxibs.

Reprinted from McKenna F and Simon L, Rapid Reference Arthritis, Mosby 2002.

gastroduodenal perforation, although this may be a contraindication even for Cox-2s,

- patients using other medications known to increase the likelihood of upper gastrointestinal adverse events, e.g., steroids and anticoagulants,
- presence of serious co-morbidity, e.g., severe heart failure, renal or liver failure, uncontrolled diabetes or uncontrolled hypertension.

Some PCTs recommend using ibuprofen plus a proton pump inhibitor instead of following NICE guidance. However:

- NICE guidance is based on evidence-based medicine and, in the case of Cox-2s, is reflective of best practice. As such, NICE guidance should be followed.
- Evidence-based medicine should be practised. At present, there is no evidence that the ibuprofen/proton pump inhibitor combination reduces perforation, ulcers and bleeds.
- There are excellent studies around the use of Cox-2s.
- Only the approaches of NICE guidance and evidence-based medicine are likely to be backed by the courts.
- Importantly, long-term studies with Cox-2s have shown a significant reduction in serious complications.

Licofelone

This is a new class of anti-inflammatory drugs designed to inhibit all of the major enzymes of the arachidonic pathway: 5-lipoxygenase (5-Lox) and Cox-1 and Cox-2. Licofelone inhibits both Lox and Cox enzymes, reducing gastrointestinal complications. A recent study showed good results in OA patients when compared with a Cox-2. Licofelone may be an alternative to Cox-2s and may offer good long-term treatment with less adverse events.

Volumes of injection fluid for different situations	
Knee	1mL steroid + 0.5mL lidocaine
CMC joint	0.25mL steroid + 0.25mL lidocaine
Flexor tendon sheath	0.25mL steroid + 0.25mL lidocaine
Shoulder	
Subacromial bursitis	1mL steroid + 1mL lidocaine
Acromioclavicular joint	0.25mL steroid + 0.25mL lidocaine
Glenohumeral capsulitis	1mL steroid + 1–9mL lidocaine (1%)
Trochanteric bursitis	1mL steroid + 4mL lidocaine

Fig. 66 Volumes of injection fluid for different situations

Other new approaches to analgesia

- Standard NSAIDs can be attached to nitric oxide (NO). The NO then attaches itself to the gastric mucosa and protects it from the harmful effects of the NSAID molecule. These drugs are now undergoing clinical trials.
- Enkephalinase inhibitors prevent degradation of endogenous opioids.
- Substance P receptor antagonists. At present there is only a topical preparation available (capsaicin). Oral drugs are now being developed.

Steroid and lidocaine injections

These injections are a widely accepted and useful mode of treating patients with many musculoskeletal conditions and are invaluable for inflammatory arthritis.

- Hydrocortisone acetate 25mg/mL, which is the least potent and shortest acting preparation. Some practitioners use this for soft-tissue problems and where there is a risk of tendon rupture, e.g., trigger finger, Achilles tendonitis or fat atrophy.
- Methylprednisolone acetate 40mg/mL (depo-medrone or depo-medrone with lidocaine), which is used extensively in primary care. It acts for longer than hydrocortisone and is said to be less potent than triamcinolone.
- Triamcinolone acetonide comes in two strengths: 10mg/mL (Adcortyl) and 40mg/mL (Kenalog). These strengths allow for varying dose regimes and practitioners' preferences.

There are no fixed rules on quantities or volumes of injection fluid. Fig. 66 is only a guide.

133

Lidocaine

A few practitioners will inject lidocaine before the steroid, usually so that the patient improves before injecting the steroid, for example, relief of a painful arc for rotator cuff tendinitis. Lidocaine may also be used to infiltrate the area to obtain greater accuracy for the following injection, for example, CMC joint injection or before injecting hyaluronan into a knee joint or injecting an acromioclavicular joint.

The strength of lidocaine (1%) is important if more than 10mL is to be injected at one session. This decreases the likelihood of central nervous system (CNS) side effects, respiratory depression or convulsions. The maximum dose of lidocaine for the average person is 200mg (10mL of 2%, 20mL of 1%). Many shoulder injections are in patients over 60 years old who may have less CNS tolerance for lidocaine.

Patient information and consent

> *Informed consent is all that is legally necessary for joint and soft-tissue injections. It may be written, oral or non-verbal*

Informed consent is all that is legally necessary for joint and soft-tissue injections. It may be written, oral or non-verbal. A signature on a consent form does not, in itself, prove that the consent is valid. It records the patient decision and that discussion has taken place. Check your local and professional society policy on this issue.

Information for patients

Practitioners usually discuss the pros and cons of injections and their side effects with patients during a consultation. It is advisable to give patients written information concerning potential problems and side effects, including information on when to seek further advice. Fig. 67 gives an example of a patient leaflet.

Repeating injections

There are no hard and fast rules, only practical guidelines:

- For repeat injections following a poor response, a 3–4-week wait seems sensible. A further injection may be appropriate for some patients with CMC joint OA and, in some cases, a course of three may be needed to give an adequate response.
- Repeat injections following a good response. Patients with knee OA may increase their mobility with pain relief for 6–8 weeks. Hopefully, a second injection will be effective for 3–4 months and further injections every 4 months will give an excellent clinical response. Some patients will require less frequent injections, especially if their mobility has helped develop the quadriceps.
- There is no rule about only injecting a joint three or four times in a year. This guidance is based on good practice. If the diagnosis is correct, it may be the only appropriate treatment.

INFORMATION FOR PATIENTS: LOCAL STEROID INJECTIONS

Injections are given to relieve swelling and pain in joints and soft tissues. The injection contains a corticosteroid which reduces inflammation and a local anaesthetic which numbs the area for a short time.

Patients may have an adverse reaction to the drugs used but this is very rare. The practitioner will ask you to wait for 20 minutes after the injection to ensure that all is well.

Patients will gain most benefit from the injection by following guidelines below:

• Rest the injected limb as much as possible for one to two days after injection.

• Avoid excessive activity for a further two weeks

Possible Side Effects

• You may experience more pain during the two days after injection. This can be relieved with paracetamol, or your normal pain killer, always following the instruction on the packet.

• It often takes several days before any improvement is noticed.

• You may experience facial flushing. Do not worry, as this usually subsides within a day or two.

• Diabetics should monitor their blood sugar as this may rise. Adjustment of diet and medication may be necessary for a few days.

• Women may experience some irregularity of the menstrual cycle after injection.

• Occasionally patients may see thinning or loss of colour of the skin at the injection site.

• *Very* rarely an injected joint can become infected: the joint becomes very painful and hot. If this occurs, contact your doctor immediately, taking this information sheet with you.

NAME .... DATE ....

Drugs used for your injection today:

Steroid .... Local anaesthetic ....

Dose .... Dose ....

Site injected ....

Steroid .... Local anaesthetic ....

Dose .... Dose ....

Site injected ....

Steroid .... Local anaesthetic ....

Dose .... Dose ....

Site injected ....

Administered by ....

If you need another appointment please contact: ....

Fig. 67 Example of a patient information leaflet about steroid injections

Hyaluronan injections

Hyaluronan is secreted by the synovial lining of a joint. It acts as a lubricant, shock absorber and joint protector and is said to have a role in repair. Hyaluronan has a high molecular weight and high viscosity. In OA, the viscosity falls and injecting hyaluronan may increase the viscosity but it is cleared rapidly from the synovial fluid. The way hyaluronan injections work is poorly understood. At present, they are used for knee OA and there are ongoing studies in hip and CMC joint OA.

"Hyaluronan is secreted by the synovial lining of a joint. It acts as a lubricant, shock absorber and joint protector and is said to have a role in repair"

135

Most preparations require a course of three to five injections into the knee joint at weekly intervals, although one preparation is one 3mL injection only (Fig. 68).

The appropriate severity of OA for these injections is still to be clarified. Hyaluronan gives poor results for patients with severe OA. Their place is probably in primary care for mild to moderate OA, to increase mobility and maintain quadriceps. Case histories show that middle- to older-aged athletes with mild OA respond remarkably well to hyaluronan injections. Response to hyaluronan injections is slow and it may take weeks before the patient sees signs of improvement. Practically, if the patient has not seen significant improvement in 3 months, they have not responded to treatment.

Hyaluronan reactions

A very small number of patients develop a severe, painful effusion after a hyaluronan injection. These require appropriate management:

Small effusion plus some discomfort

Advise patients to take their pain medication for the discomfort and to use an ice pack wrapped in a towel for 10–20 minutes, as necessary.

Severe discomfort plus an effusion

These patients may have a tense knee and even though the effusion contains only approximately 20mL, it plays a large part in the discomfort and pain. Pain relief on removing the fluid is immediate and excellent. The fluid is usually straw coloured; if not, it should be sent for culture to exclude infection: this is one differential diagnosis; the other is a ruptured Baker's cyst.

Fig. 68 Hyaluronan preparations for osteoarthritic knees

Drug	Dose	Regimen
Durolane (synthetic)	3mL	As a single intra-articular injection. Repeat after 6 months prn.
Hyalgan (avian)	2mL	Weekly intra-articular injections for a total of 5 injections. Repeat courses after 6 months prn.
Synvisc (avian)	2mL	Weekly intra-articular injections for a total of 3 injections. Maximum of 6 injections in 6 months.
Ostenil (synthetic)	2mL	Weekly intra-articular injections for up to 5 injections. Repeat courses at 6 months prn.

Patients who do well are those with mild to moderate OA and who are still relatively active, i.e., they have a physical activity or hobby such as dog walking, hiking, etc.

Large effusion with knee pain

Large effusions should be drained to give immediate pain relief. A sample should be sent for culture to exclude infection. The fluid is usually straw coloured and sterile. If the effusion recurs, aspiration should be repeated. Do not delay, as the rapid re-accumulation of fluid can cause severe discomfort and pain. NSAIDs/Cox-2s do not appear to stop the accumulation of fluid but they do give good pain relief. Aspiration gives the best relief. Injecting steroid after aspiration does not appear to prevent the re-accumulation of fluid. Sometimes, aspiration is necessary on 3 successive days.

❝Large effusions should be drained to give immediate pain relief. A sample should be sent for culture to exclude infection ❞

Pseudo-infection effusion with knee pain

This effusion is rarely seen but, when it does occur, causes great anxiety for both patient and doctor. There is little difference in the pain and discomfort caused in comparison to the large, straw-coloured effusion but the fluid looks like frank pus, i.e., yellow/grey/green. The knee is warm but not excessively so. The patient has severe knee pain but is not ill or febrile. The fluid should be sent for culture and microscopy but, importantly, the patient should not be treated for infection solely on a laboratory report of macrophages. Treating inappropriately with an antibiotic such as gentamicin may lead to greater side effects than those caused by the hyaluronan. Removing the fluid gives good pain relief. The joint does not require washout or surgical debridement. Medical staff must be informed about these reactions to hyaluronan otherwise there is a risk of inappropriate treatment, causing the patient further distress.

Further courses of hyaluronan

A good response to a course of hyaluronan may give increased mobility and pain relief for 4–18 months. Courses can be repeated.

Glucosamine

Glucosamine, a complex amino sugar, is a normal constituent of the glycosaminoglycans that are found in cartilage matrix and synovial fluid. As an oral preparation, it is absorbed and distributed to the joint tissues.

Trials evidence

Studies have raised great interest in this compound. In a double-blind RCT with 3 years' follow-up, 212 patients with mild to moderate knee OA received placebo or glucosamine 1500mg daily. The primary outcome measure for structural change was the mean joint space width of the medial compartment of the tibiofemoral joint measured radiologically using a standard technique. For OA symptoms, the primary outcome measure was the visual analogue WOMAC scale (appendix 5). The results were encouraging: there was progressive narrowing of the joint space in the placebo group (106 patients) but no significant loss of joint space in the treatment arm (106 patients). WOMAC scores showed improvement in the glucosamine arm and slight worsening in the placebo arm. Safety and early withdrawal were the same for the two groups. These results need confirming with a larger group and longer follow up.

In another, 6-month RCT of 80 patients with knee OA, patients continued taking their analgesics or NSAIDs and were encouraged not to change doses or preparations during the study. The patient's global assessment of pain in the affected knee was the primary outcome. Analysis showed no difference between the glucosamine and placebo arms, although there was a small but statistically significant improvement in knee flexion. The conclusion was that glucosamine was no more effective than placebo in modifying pain in patients with a wide range of pain severity.

Why the difference between these two studies?
- The second study included patients with more severe OA (by X-ray and symptoms) than the first. Glucosamine may be indicated in early disease.
- The second study was small; a larger study may give different results.

A large, long-term study is being undertaken by the US National Institutes of Health (NIH). It is expected that this will answer the debate.

Referral and surgical interventions

Historically, primary care has referred the majority of MSK problems, excluding inflammatory cases, to orthopaedic surgeons (Fig. 69). The change in emphasis to fund and administer more of the NHS via primary care is producing many changes, hopefully for the benefit of patients. One major change is the introduction of GPwSI in MSK. These doctors are developing different models of care and work in different localities, such as:

Historically, primary care has referred the majority of MSK problems, excluding inflammatory cases, to orthopaedic surgeons

- GP surgeries,
- within a multidisciplinary team including physiotherapists, podiatrists and sometimes occupational therapists with back up from rheumatologists, plastic surgeons and orthopaedic surgeons,
- alongside secondary care in a hospital.

It is expected that, given time, research projects will produce an evidence base, which is long overdue. The process has started, with designated research practices with appropriate funding and an academic and management structure.

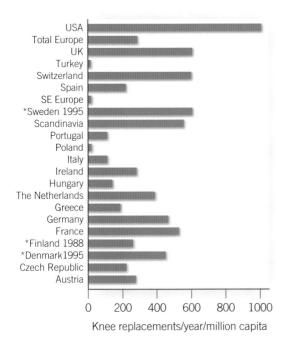

Fig. 69 Annual knee replacement rates for OA are increasing. However, there is no evidence that knee replacement for severe knee OA is over-utilized. In general, at least two-thirds of patients who receive replacement knees are women. Mean age at arthroplasty is about 70 years. More than 80% of knee replacements are for OA. Reprinted from http://www.move.uk.net/basic_04.jsp. *Data found in the literature.

Most non-inflammatory musculoskeletal patients can be managed in primary care, either by the GP, a community physiotherapist or a GPwSI and the multidisciplinary team. Only patients who require, and are willing to undergo, surgery should be referred to an orthopaedic surgeon.

Meniscal and meniscectomy problems

- Sports personnel, especially football players, risk knee injuries.
- Total meniscectomy causes a high incidence of OA in the operated knee.
- There is also an increased incidence in the non-operated knee.
- Partial meniscectomy leads to the development of OA in 50% of patients.
- The lateral meniscus is less often damaged and operated upon. If it is removed, there is an even greater risk of OA developing compared to medial meniscectomy.
- Elite athletes, especially footballers who may have associated cruciate ligament damage, have the greatest risk of developing OA after knee operations.

" Most non-inflammatory musculoskeletal patients can be managed in primary care, either by the GP, a community physiotherapist or a GPwSI and the multidisciplinary team "

139

> *Patients with OA who develop sudden knee pain with an effusion that does not settle, as in an OA flare, have probably sustained a meniscal injury from a twisting injury/activity*

- Patients with OA who develop sudden knee pain with an effusion that does not settle, as in an OA flare, have probably sustained a meniscal injury from a twisting injury/activity.

Injuries, effusions and washouts

- Injuries and fractures involving joint surfaces are likely to lead to OA in later life. If repair does not produce normal alignment, the joint is stressed.
- Joints that are unstable or move too far, as occurs in hypermobility, are more likely to develop OA.
- A knee becomes unstable if there is major cruciate damage. These joints degenerate even if there is no meniscal damage.
- The best protection for all joints, especially knees, is to develop the muscles around the joint.
- With advancing years, muscles become weaker and joints less stable and so more prone to injury that may lead to OA or accelerate the OA process.
- A knee effusion, even relatively small, will cause rapid wasting of the quadriceps.
- Drainage of an effusion will give pain relief and help mobility. In practice, removal of more than 5mL of synovial fluid will give immediate pain relief, encouraging mobility.
- Traumatic effusions should be aspirated to check for blood, which signifies greater, usually cruciate, damage. If there is blood, the knee will feel boggy and warm. If the knee is tense, severe pain will also be experienced.
- Synovial effusions are relatively common in OA, signifying cartilage damage. The size of the effusion varies from minimal to extremely large. Extremely large effusions are seen in severely damaged knees and require secondary referral if they recur. The patient usually requires a new knee joint but if the co-morbidity excludes this solution, a medical synovectomy using yttrium, or similar compound, may be another option.
- Arthroscopic surgery can debride joints, perform meniscectomies and repair ACLs.

Is debridement worthwhile?

In most patients, the answer is no. Primary care staff need to be highly selective when referring patients for debridement as it is not a panacea. A recent trial divided patients into three groups of 60 patients: placebo, lavage and debridement.

- All patients were < 75 years and fulfilled ACR criteria for OA.

> *Primary care staff need to be highly selective when referring patients for debridement as it is not a panacea*

- Patients had a pain score of ≥ 40 mm on a 100mm visual analogue scale.
- Follow-up was for 2 years.
- There was no difference in outcome between the three groups.

Orthopaedic surgeons, arthroplasty and osteotomy

Surgeons wish to see patients who require operation. The criteria for hips and knees is patients who can't sleep, can't walk or can't work. Pain, not the X-ray grade, is the most important parameter for referral and operation. Evidence suggests that if the pain becomes too severe or chronic, postoperative results are poor as the chronic pain persists. Patient-relevant outcomes after total hip replacement for OA show that a higher age and more pain preoperatively predict a poor outcome.

> *Surgeons wish to see patients who require operation. The criteria for hips and knees is patients who can't sleep, can't walk or can't work*

Arthroplasty outcomes

- Hip and knee arthroplasties have been a resounding success.
- Shoulder arthroplasty does not improve movement function but does relieve pain.
- Ankle arthroplasty is good for RA but results in OA are awaited.
- Small-joint arthroplasties are not as successful as large-joint surgery.
- Severe thumb and big-toe OA respond better to arthrodesis (joint fusion) or osteotomy than arthroplasty.

Revision rates and complications of arthroplasties

- Arthroplasties give a success rate of 90% at 10 years and 75% are functioning well at 15 years.
- The Swedish National Arthroplasty Register for hips gives a revision rate for infection of 0.6% at 10 years. Half of these are due to intra-operative contamination and the other half are due to haematogenous spread from the urinary tract, lungs, gall bladder or dental abscess (Fig. 70).
- Loosening is the commonest cause of revision (about 10% at 10 years).
- The most common complication is deep vein thrombosis (in 10% of patients); 1% of patients suffer a pulmonary embolism.

The following factors help to reduce arthroplasty complications:

- early mobilization,
- continually improving surgical techniques,
- prophylactic anticoagulation,
- peri-operative antibiotics,
- critical appraisal trials of new joint design,
- registers to collate statistics, both local and national,
- informing patients and carers improves outcomes.

> *Arthroplasties give a success rate of 90% at 10 years and 75% are functioning well at 15 years*

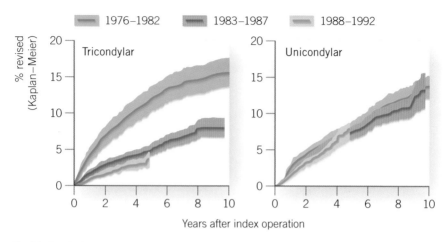

Fig. 70 Prosthetic revision rates. Reprinted from Brandt et al. Acta Orthop Scand 1994;65:375–88.

Problems with arthroplasties

What are the signs of loosening?

* increasing pain,
* instability or increasing lack of confidence on walking,
* a lucent line seen on X-ray.

What are the signs of infection?

* onset of new pain or a change in character of the pain,
* deep pain on weight bearing,
* clinical signs of inflammation (temperature, sweating, febrile),
* site of infection,
* raised ESR and CRP.

> *Informing patients and carers improves outcomes*

Patient information

* Informing patients and carers improves outcomes.
* Realistic, attainable goals should be set for each patient.
* Fully explain the purpose and goals of the patient exercise regime.
* The patient must be able to undertake the exercises.
* Patients require ongoing reassurance and encouragement. Many discontinue the exercises and do not gain full benefit from the operation.
* Social and carer support for recovery at home must be adequate.
* Patients and carers will need advice on:
  – what to do,
  – what not to do,
  – how to cope,
  – when to seek help and advice. Many hospitals have a helpline for patients, carers and doctors.

Fig. 71 Wedge resection

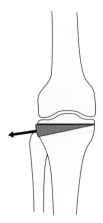

- Potential problems and pitfalls, both common and specific, should be explained to the patient and carer.
- Timescales of progress must be explained, e.g., driving a car is permissible after 6 weeks, physical improvements can continue for up to 1–2 years.
- If the joint becomes painful and swollen, apply ice and temporarily decrease the amount of exercise.
- Caution: prolonged immobilization increases the risk of postoperative complications by causing muscle atrophy, decreasing the range of movements and hence lowering goals.

Osteotomy

Osteotomy corrects bad joint alignment and transfers the stresses on the damaged portion of a joint to areas with more articular cartilage. For a knee, this requires a wedge of bone being removed from the less damaged side (Fig. 71).

- Careful selection of patients is required as this operation is demanding mentally and physically.
- The results are not as good as those for arthroplasty.
- Osteotomy should be considered for patients with severe pain and high activity demands, e.g., farmers wishing to continue active work or people involved in high-activity leisure pursuits such as hill walking or skiing. They should have an activity age of 60 years or less.

Osteoporosis and osteomalacia
Osteoporosis

Osteoporosis, the most common disease affecting bone, is defined as reduced bone mass (osteopenia) and increased fragility to an extent sufficient to result in fractures on minimal trauma.

> *Osteoporotic hip fractures have a high mortality rate and, from a public health standpoint, an even higher morbidity because of the number of people that require residential care*

> *Vertebral osteoporosis usually causes asymptomatic compression fractures in people aged over 70 years. Patients develop kyphosis and some restriction of activities but have little or no pain*

> *Hypovitaminosis D osteopathy, and even frank osteomalacia, may occur in immigrant women who are dark skinned, have inadequate exposure to sunlight, are vegetarians and eat chapattis*

- Fractures usually occur when bone mass is 30–40% below normal values, but osteoporosis is a multifactorial disease, not simply ageing.
- Fractures most frequently affect the spine, hip and wrist.
- Osteoporosis mostly affects women but, as the population ages, it is increasingly becoming a public health issue in both sexes.
- Osteoporotic hip fractures have a high mortality rate and, from a public health standpoint, an even higher morbidity because of the number of people that require residential care.

Osteoporosis is a large enough subject for a book to itself. However, there is a great deal that the primary care team can achieve. All practices should be involved in prevention and earlier intervention for this potentially catastrophic disease. The Primary Care Rheumatology Society has produced minimum standard guidelines that meet these criteria. Importantly, these include the facts and figures concerning the questions from, and information that is often requested by, patients (see appendix 4).

Vertebral osteoporosis

Vertebral osteoporosis usually causes asymptomatic compression fractures in people aged over 70 years. Patients develop kyphosis and some restriction of activities but have little or no pain. If the patient lives long enough, pain may arise from damaged apophyseal joints but spinal cord problems are rare. Patients rarely have so much kyphosis/compression that the ribs rest on the iliac crests, which can cause considerable pain.

Corticosteroids and osteoporosis

Most patients taking corticosteroids have not been evaluated or treated for their osteoporosis risk. The majority of these patients are under GP care and, as stated in the PCR Minimum Standard Guidelines, their risk should be assessed.

Patients aged at least 65 years who start corticosteroids should immediately be prescribed treatment for osteoporosis prevention. PMR is the classic diagnosis where prevention is recommended at the start of treatment (see appendix 4 page 180).

Osteomalacia

Osteomalacia is defined as a defect of skeletal mineralization due to vitamin D deficiency. Hypovitaminosis D osteopathy, and even frank osteomalacia, may occur in immigrant women who are dark skinned, have inadequate exposure to sunlight, are vegetarians and eat chapattis. They present with widespread musculoskeletal pain and bony tenderness and may be diagnosed as suffering from fibromyalgia. The diagnosis is

based on a low serum vitamin D and response to vitamin D supplements. The clinical features include:
- bone pain, often vague and poorly localized in the axial skeleton, especially in the pubic rami and ribs,
- bone tenderness,
- possible proximal myopathy with weakness causing a waddling gait,
- spontaneous fractures.

Diagnosis is confirmed by:
- blood tests: show low serum calcium, phosphorus and vitamin D levels and a high alkaline phosphatase,
- X-rays may show "looser's zones",
- bone biopsy: will confirm the diagnosis but is rarely necessary.

Future trends in musculoskeletal medicine

It is always difficult to predict future trends. Our understanding of the pathogenesis of musculoskeletal disorders is increasing at an exponential rate. This increased knowledge will have an impact on the management of these conditions both in primary and secondary care. Some of the newer managements will undoubtedly entail the use of drugs or other therapies with powerful effects, both for good and for ill, in which case they would be used in secondary care but in partnership with primary care physicians.

66 Our understanding of the pathogenesis of musculoskeletal disorders is increasing at an exponential rate 99

Referral guidelines

Referral guidelines, which have already been developed in some PCTs, are to be welcomed as they will reflect local circumstances and facilities. However, national referral guidelines can also be extremely useful, particularly if they can be audited so that one can measure the degree to which they are being followed. Some of the information contained in this book could be used to develop referral guidelines in conjunction with the local rheumatologist.

66 Referral guidelines are to be welcomed as they will reflect local circumstances and facilities 99

Electronic appointments

An advantage of referral guidelines is that they can be easily adapted so that electronic appointments can be made directly from primary care to the local rheumatology department. An additional advantage of electronic referral, apart from the obvious ones of bypassing delays in the postal system and reducing the handling and storage of paper, is that red and yellow flags can be inserted at appropriate places. This can alert the referring physician to any problems that might require more urgent attention or to additional investigations that need to be done before consultation, thus encouraging cost-effective use of resources

66 An additional advantage of electronic referral is that red and yellow flags can be inserted at appropriate places 99

145

and saving time. Some Trusts have already implemented electronic referral, at least on a trial basis.

Shared care

> *Increasingly, shared care protocols have been and are being developed between secondary and primary care*

Increasingly, shared care protocols have been and are being developed between secondary and primary care. These are inevitable developments, as with the shortage of rheumatologists, the primary care physician has a major responsibility in following up his/her patients in collaboration with the rheumatologist. However, there must be a clear line of management so that the patient does not fall uncomfortably between two stools.

Rheumatology in primary care

It seems unlikely that there will be a very large expansion in the number of consultant rheumatologists in the near future. Since primary care physicians already see the bulk of musculoskeletal conditions, it is logical that more of them should be trained to have the appropriate level of expertise and skill within the community. The vast majority of patients being followed by consultant rheumatologists have inflammatory diseases, mostly RA. It may be that with fewer referrals to rheumatologists, there may be a greater emphasis on the treatment of serious but common conditions such as OA. There needs to be imaginative interaction between the primary and the secondary care sectors with the development of triage clinics, manned by physiotherapists or nurses who can sort through problems and make the appropriate referral to either primary or secondary care: back pain is being triaged in several centres in this cost-effective way.

> *There needs to be imaginative interaction between the primary and the secondary care sectors*

Targeted therapies

This is undoubtedly the most exciting area of development in rheumatology today and for the foreseeable future. We are familiar with targeted therapies in the drugs that interfere with and/or augment particular biochemical pathways. For example, the variety of pharmacological interventions that act at different levels to control hypertension.

Until recently, targeted therapies were not available for many rheumatological diseases. Exceptions included gout, in which allopurinol specifically inhibits enzyme pathways that lead to the production of uric acid. Serious and complex diseases such as RA and SLE did not have such clearly defined targets. The situation has changed dramatically over the last 2 years, due to the introduction of targeted RA therapies directed at inhibiting TNFα. These treatments may also be applied to other diseases such as ankylosing spondylitis and SLE.

Targeted therapies may take the form of either a protein (biologic therapy) or classic low-molecular-weight drugs active by mouth.

There are many targeted therapies in the pipeline for the treatment of RA. Some are aimed at immune regulatory cells or pathways. One such treatment is directed at killing the B-cells that make RF by infusion of an anti-B-cell monoclonal antibody, rituximab. This treatment appears to be well tolerated and to improve the disease for a year or more without additional treatment. The outcome of large Phase III studies is eagerly awaited. Another treatment is based on the administration of a low-molecular-weight, orally active drug that inhibits the activity of a protein called p38. This is crucially involved in the signalling pathways that lead to the secretion of inflammatory cytokines.

❝This is undoubtedly the most exciting area of development in rheumatology today and for the foreseeable future❞

Case study 1
Rheumatoid arthritis

History

Six months ago, 65-year-old Mr A. developed left mid foot pain which he thought was due to excessive walking: he plays golf four times a week. A month later, he developed stiffness in his left shoulder and arm, pain in the right wrist and stiffness in his legs and hips. He was prescribed indomethacin and his condition improved. Three months ago, his problems returned, this time affecting his shoulder and pelvic girdles. There was some stiffness of the small joints of his hands and he complained of increasing weakness. A clinical diagnosis of PMR was made. He was started on prednisolone 7.5mg each morning, which brought about a marked improvement. After 3 weeks, prednisolone was reduced to 5mg daily. At this time, plasma viscosity (PV) was 1.84 and RF was 138 IU (normal, 0–20).

Six weeks after starting on prednisolone, when his dose was reduced to 2.5mg/5mg on alternate days, his symptoms returned with a vengeance. He was much stiffer and in more pain than previously and unable to turn over in bed. The stiffness lasted all morning and returned after tea. He was becoming increasingly depressed about his poor quality of life and especially about not being able to play golf. He complained of two new problems, swelling of the left calf and a generalized itch. The itch was thought to be caused by an enzyme-based washing powder and he was advised to change to a sensitive skin type and to stop using soft rinse.

He was commenced on a higher dose of prednisolone (10mg). An urgent appointment was requested and a week later he saw a consultant rheumatologist.

> *Six weeks after starting on prednisolone, when his dose was reduced to 2.5mg/5mg on alternate days, his symptoms returned with a vengeance*

Examination

The general examination was unremarkable, with a blood pressure of 140/70mmHg and no myopathy or lymphadenopathy. Locomotor examination showed reduced flexion/extension of both wrists, synovitis of the index and middle finger MCP joints, a 10-degree loss of extension in both elbows, left shoulder stiffness, left popliteal fullness, a swollen left calf and normal ankles and feet. PV was 1.90 and RF was 171 IU.

Diagnosis

Rheumatoid arthritis was diagnosed, with probable ruptured Baker's cyst in the left calf. Ultrasound showed no evidence of deep vein thrombosis, only Baker's cyst.

Management

The patient received diclofenac 75mg, one tablet twice daily, prednisolone 7.5mg daily and sulphasalazine 500mg daily, increasing weekly to 2g daily. A monitoring regime was instigated. At follow-up 4 months later, the patient was improving and had a better quality of life; he was able to play some golf again. At this time, the prednisolone dose was reduced to 5mg daily and sulphasalazine was increased to 3g daily.

Practical points

- PMR is essentially a diagnosis of exclusion.
- Initial good response to small doses of steroids was impressive but did not last. Larger doses may have delayed the correct diagnosis.
- Perhaps more attention should have been given to the hand joint problems.
- A telephone call to a rheumatologist certainly benefited Mr A.
- A high RF indicated a likely diagnosis in this patient with hand joint problems, but in practice this is not foolproof (see **arc** website, Hands On, PMR, case history, where the diagnosis was PMR and not rheumatoid arthritis with a RF of 382).

❝PMR is essentially a diagnosis of exclusion❞

❝Perhaps more attention should have been given to the hand joint problems❞

Case study 2
Achilles tendonitis

History

This 57-year-old market trader spends around 10 hours a day standing at a stall in all weathers. She is very overweight and has been so most of her life. She previously had a thyroidectomy and takes thyroxine. She is not a diabetic. She nearly always wears slip on shoes. She presented with pain in her left heel.

Examination

She had pain on palpation of her Achilles tendon, which was more tender down the lateral border. The tendon was diffusely thickened but not red.

Diagnosis

Left Achilles tendonitis.

Management

The patient was given a 3-month course of depo-medrone 0.5mL + 1mL lignocaine into the paratendon, with one injection/month. She was asked to massage the tendon after taking a shower or a bath. This treatment gave only short-term pain relief of 10 days or less. The patient was then supplied with sorbothane $3/_4$ arch cushions to be worn in her shoes and her slippers. She was advised not to walk around in bare feet, to perform stretching exercises and to continue to massage her Achilles tendon. The insoles gave pain relief and she continued to wear them for almost 1 year before she was completely pain free. She did massage her tendon but did not do the stretching exercises as she said that she had to be up very early to set out her market stall. She has not lost weight. Two years later, she no longer wears insoles but is still pain free.

❝ The insoles gave pain relief and she continued to wear them for almost 1 year before she was completely pain free ❞

❝ She did not need to lose weight for the insoles to allow/promote healing ❞

Practical points

- Steroid injections only give temporary relief.
- Wearing $3/_4$ arch cushions was an attainable goal for pain relief and for correcting the biomechanical problems.
- Stretching exercises was a goal too far, but if performed may have reduced the recovery time (for exercises see appendix 5 page 184).
- She did not need to lose weight for the insoles to allow/promote healing.

Case study 3
Ankylosing spondylitis

History

Mr M. spent many years in the army, representing the army in weight lifting, for which he spent a good deal of time training. After leaving the army he joined the building trade. He retired aged 60 years and over the past 2 years has had increasing difficulty with his back. He applied for a disability allowance but this was refused. A month ago he visited his general practitioner because he was finding it more and more difficult to put his socks and trousers on. His back movements were very restricted; there was little forward flexion and his hands were only able to reach as far as his knees. He was sent for X-ray and the report stated: "Lumbar Spine: There is bilateral sacroiliitis present. The facet joints are also abnormal with a pattern that looks more typical of inflammatory spondylitis than simple facet osteoarthritis. More superior there is prominent paraspinal osteophytosis, which is not typical of ankylosing spondylitis. Is there a history of psoriasis? Suggest rheumatology opinion." He was referred to a rheumatologist.

Examination

All neck movements were restricted, especially lateral flexion. Head extension was almost zero. There was minimal spinal rotation, and spinal flexion was really all from the pelvis. There was no peripheral synovitis (hand joints were normal), but there was mild to moderate osteoarthritis of the right knee. There was pain on "springing" sacroiliac joints.

Diagnosis

Ankylosing spondylitis.

Management

The patient received etoricoxib 120mg daily, sulphasalazine 1000mg daily for 10 days then twice daily (monitoring as per protocol). He was referred for physiotherapy with a request to occupational therapy to perform a home assessment for aids and appliances.

"There was minimal spinal rotation, and spinal flexion was really all from the pelvis. There was no peripheral synovitis (hand joints were normal), but there was mild to moderate osteoarthritis of the right knee"

Practical points

- Always ask about psoriasis or a family history of psoriasis or inflammatory joint disease, which can all be linked to such X-ray changes.

"There is no evidence that sulphasalazine or methotrexate have any effect on spinal disease, only on peripheral arthritis"

- There is no evidence that sulphasalazine or methotrexate have any effect on spinal disease, only on peripheral arthritis. Only anti-TNF has been shown to suppress spinal disease and improve pain, morning stiffness and spinal mobility.

- His previous occupation appeared to give Mr M. enough natural physiotherapy. It is possible this man had hypermobility in addition to his physical fitness to account for the delay in diagnosis.

- X-rays may help in patients who present with an atypical history of back pain.

- Non-pharmacological treatments are particularly important for patients with ankylosing spondylitis.

- Etoricoxib has been shown to be powerful in relieving pain and is warranted for patients with ankylosing spondylitis (phenylbutazone is no longer available).

- He will require a letter from his physician to help him appeal against the Disability Living Allowance decision.

"This delay in diagnosis is unusual in a male. The diagnosis in females may be delayed for 10 years compared to the diagnosis in males"

- This delay in diagnosis is unusual in a male. The diagnosis in females may be delayed for 10 years compared to the diagnosis in males.

Case study 4
Rheumatoid arthritis

A 35-year-old female financial accountant consulted her general practitioner with swollen and sore feet. Pain and stiffness in the mornings eased during the day. Over the next several weeks, other joints were involved including the knees, the elbows, the wrists and the small joints of the hands, with prolonged early morning stiffness and pain in the joints and waking up in the middle of the night. Tests showed a positive rheumatoid factor and an elevated sedimentation rate. She was diagnosed as having rheumatoid arthritis. Over the next 10 years, she had a variety of treatments including hydroxychloroquine and intra-muscular gold, which were ineffective, azathioprine, which produced severe nausea and had to be discontinued, and sulphasalazine, which induced erythema multiforme. Methotrexate produced a partial response with the DAS falling from 6.5 to 4.3, but was discontinued because she wished to have a family. Penicillamine to a maximum of 1g at night elicited no response whatsoever. Her attempts at having a baby having failed on several attempts and because the activity of the rheumatoid arthritis worsened (DAS 5.8), she decided to have more effective therapy. She was given an anti-TNF biologic against a background of 15mg methotrexate weekly. Within 3 months, she went into remission with a Disease Activity Score of 2.2. At this level of disease activity, her joint damage is slowed and even halted. She has been registered on the British Society of Rheumatology Biologics Register.

Comment

This is an example of a patient who failed all disease-modifying therapy either because of lack of efficacy or toxicity. The NICE Guidelines for anti-TNFα biologic therapy for rheumatoid arthritis are:

- failure of two or more DMARDs,
- DAS > 5.1,
- patient enrolled on the British Society of Rheumatology Biologics Register, which monitors medium- and long-term toxicity and efficacy,
- therapy should be withdrawn for severe drug-related toxicity or lack of efficacy at 6 months.

" Therapy should be withdrawn for severe drug–related toxicity or lack of efficacy at 6 months "

Non-steroidal anti-inflammatory agents (NSAIDs)

Drug	Format	Trade name	Preparation	Strength	Doses used in arthritis (adult)	Comments	Side effects
Aceclofenac	Oral	Preservex	Tablet	100mg	100mg 2 times/d	Take with or after food	Gastrointestinal discomfort, nausea, diarrhoea; gastrointestinal bleeding and ulceration; hypersensitivity reactions; headache, dizziness, vertigo, hearing disturbances
Acemetacin	Oral	Emflex	Capsule	60mg	60mg 2-3 times/d	Glycolic acid ester of indometacin; take with or after food	Gastrointestinal discomfort, nausea, diarrhoea; gastrointestinal bleeding and ulceration; hypersensitivity reactions; headache, dizziness, vertigo, hearing disturbances
Azapropazone	Oral	Rheumox	Capsule Tablet	300mg 600mg	300-600mg 2-4 times/d (max. 1.2g/d); elderly max. 300mg 2 times/d	Use restricted to rheumatoid arthritis when other NSAIDs have failed; avoid direct exposure to sunlight or use sunblock; take with or after food	Gastrointestinal discomfort, nausea, diarrhoea; gastrointestinal bleeding and ulceration (may be severe); hypersensitivity reactions (may be severe); headache, dizziness, vertigo, hearing disturbances; photosensitivity reactions
Dexketoprofen	Oral	Keral	Tablet	25mg	12.5-25mg 3-4 times daily (max. 75mg/d); elderly max. 50mg/d	Isomer of ketoprofen; used for short term treatment of pain; take with or after food	Gastrointestinal discomfort, nausea, diarrhoea; gastrointestinal bleeding and ulceration; hypersensitivity reactions; headache, dizziness, vertigo, hearing disturbances
Diclofenac sodium	Oral	Diclomax SR	M/R capsule	75mg	75-150mg 1-2 times/d (max. 150mg)	Take with or after food	Gastrointestinal discomfort, nausea, diarrhoea; gastrointestinal bleeding and ulceration; hypersensitivity reactions; headache, dizziness, vertigo, hearing disturbances
		Diclomax Retard	M/R capsule	100mg	100mg/d		
		Motifene	M/R E/C capsule	75mg	75mg 1-2 times/d		
		Voltarol	Tablet	25mg, 50mg	75-150mg/d		
		Voltarol SR	M/R tablet	75mg	75mg 1-2 times/d		
		Voltarol Retard	M/R tablet	100mg	100mg/d		

Non-steroidal anti-inflammatory agents (NSAIDs)

Drug	Format	Trade name	Preparation	Strength	Doses used in arthritis (adult)	Comments	Side effects
Diclofenac sodium (cont'd)	Oral	Arthrotec	Tablet	50mg, 75mg (with misoprostol 200mcg)	1 tablet 2-3 times/d	Used as prophylaxis against NSAID-induced gastroduodenal ulceration; contraindicated in pregnant women and women planning a pregnancy	
	Topical	Voltarol	Emulgel	1%	Apply 3-4 times/d		Hypersensitivity reactions
	Rectal	Voltarol	Suppository	12.5mg, 25mg, 50mg, 100mg	75-100mg/d in divided doses		Rectal irritation and occasional bleeding
Diflunisal	Oral	Dolobid	Tablet	250mg, 500mg	500-1000mg 1-2 times/d (max. 1000mg)	Take with or after food	Gastrointestinal discomfort, nausea, diarrhoea; gastrointestinal bleeding and ulceration; hypersensitivity reactions; headache, dizziness, vertigo, hearing disturbances
Etodolac	Oral	Lodine SR	M/R tablet	600mg	600mg/d	Take with or after food	Gastrointestinal discomfort, nausea, diarrhoea; gastrointestinal bleeding and ulceration; hypersensitivity reactions; headache, dizziness, vertigo, hearing disturbances
Felbinac	Topical	Traxam	Foam, gel	3%	Apply 2-4 times/d	Active metabolite of fenbufen	Hypersensitivity reactions
Fenbufen	Oral	Lederfen	Capsule	300mg	300mg mane/ 600mg nocte	Take with or after food	Gastrointestinal discomfort, nausea, diarrhoea; gastrointestinal bleeding and ulceration; hypersensitivity reactions (high risk); headache, dizziness, vertigo, hearing disturbances; erythema multiforme; Stevens-Johnson syndrome
			Tablet	300mg, 450mg	450mg 2 times/d		
Fenoprofen	Oral	Fenopron	Tablet	300mg, 600mg	300-600mg 3-4 times/d (max. 3g/d)	Take with or after food	Gastrointestinal discomfort, nausea, diarrhoea; gastrointestinal bleeding and ulceration; hypersensitivity reactions; headache, dizziness, vertigo, hearing disturbances

Non-steroidal anti-inflammatory agents (NSAIDs)

Drug	Format	Trade name	Preparation	Strength	Doses used in arthritis (adult)	Comments	Side effects
Flurbiprofen	Oral	Froben	Tablet	50mg, 100mg	150-200mg/d in divided doses	Take with or after food	Gastrointestinal discomfort, nausea, diarrhoea; gastrointestinal bleeding and ulceration; hypersensitivity reactions; headache, dizziness, vertigo, hearing disturbances
		Froben SR	Capsule	200mg	200mg/d		
	Rectal	Froben	Suppository	100mg	100-200mg/d in divided doses		Rectal irritation and occasional bleeding
Ibuprofen	Oral	Brufen	Tablet	200mg, 400mg, 600mg	1200-1800mg in 3-4 divided doses (max. 2400mg/d)	Take with or after food	Gastrointestinal discomfort, nausea, diarrhoea; gastrointestinal bleeding and ulceration; hypersensitivity reactions; headache, dizziness, vertigo, hearing disturbances
		Brufen	Syrup	100mg/5ml	1200-1800mg in 3-4 divided doses (max. 2400mg/d)		
		Brufen Retard	M/R tablet	800mg	1600mg/d		
		Fenbid	Spansule	300mg	300-900mg 2 times/d		
		Codafen Continuus	M/R tablet	300mg (with codeine 20mg)	1-2 tablets 2 times/d		
	Topical	Ibugel	Gel	5%, 10%	Apply 3-4 times/d		Hypersensitivity reactions
Indometacin	Oral	Indocid	Capsule	25mg, 50mg	50-200mg/d in divided doses	Caution patients about dizziness if driving; take with or after food	Gastrointestinal discomfort, nausea, diarrhoea (frequent); gastrointestinal bleeding and ulceration; hypersensitivity reactions; headache, dizziness and light-headedness, vertigo, hearing disturbances
		Indocid R	M/R capsule	75mg	75mg 1-2 times/d		
		Flexin	M/R tablet	25mg, 50mg, 75mg	25-200mg/d in divided doses		
	Rectal	Indocid	Suppository	100mg	100mg 1-2 times/d		

Non-steroidal anti-inflammatory agents (NSAIDs)

Drug	Format	Trade name	Preparation	Strength	Doses used in arthritis (adult)	Comments	Side effects
Ketoprofen	Topical	Oruvail, Powergel	Gel	2.5%	Apply 2-4 times/d		Hypersensitivity reactions
Lornoxicam	Oral	Xefo	Tablet	4mg, 8mg	12mg/d in divided doses	Take with or after food	Gastrointestinal discomfort, nausea, diarrhoea; gastrointestinal bleeding and ulceration; hypersensitivity reactions; headache, dizziness, vertigo, hearing disturbances
Mefenamic acid	Oral	Ponstan	Capsule	250mg	500mg 3 times/d	Take with or after food	Gastrointestinal discomfort, nausea, diarrhoea; gastrointestinal bleeding and ulceration; hypersensitivity reactions; headache, dizziness, vertigo, hearing disturbances
		Ponstan Forte	Tablet	500mg			
Meloxicam	Oral	Mobic	Tablet	7.5mg, 15mg	7.5-15mg/d (elderly 7.5mg/d)	Take with or after food; avoid rectal administration in proctitis or haemorrhoids	Gastrointestinal discomfort, nausea, diarrhoea; gastrointestinal bleeding and ulceration; hypersensitivity reactions; headache, dizziness, vertigo, hearing disturbances
	Rectal	Mobic	Suppository	7.5mg			Rectal irritation and occasional bleeding
Meclofenamate sodium	Oral	Meclomen	Capsule	50mg	50mg 4-6 times/d (max 400mg/d)	Take with or after food	Gastrointestinal discomfort, nausea, diarrhoea; gastrointestinal bleeding and ulceration; hypersensitivity reactions; headache, dizziness, vertigo, hearing disturbances
Nabumetone	Oral	Relifex	Tablet	500mg	1000-2000mg/d in divided doses	Take with or after food	Gastrointestinal discomfort, nausea, diarrhoea; gastrointestinal bleeding and ulceration; hypersensitivity reactions; headache, dizziness, vertigo, hearing disturbances
Naproxen	Oral	Naprosyn	Tablet; E/C tablet	250mg, 375mg, 500mg	250-500mg 2 times/d	Take with or after food	Gastrointestinal discomfort, nausea, diarrhoea; gastrointestinal bleeding and ulceration; hypersensitivity reactions; headache, dizziness, vertigo, hearing disturbances
		Naprosyn	Suspension	125mg/5ml	250-500mg 2 times/d		
		Naprosyn S/R	Tablet	500mg	500-1000mg/d		
		Synflex	Tablet	275mg	550mg 2 times/d		

Non-steroidal anti-inflammatory agents (NSAIDs)

Drug	Format	Trade name	Preparation	Strength	Doses used in arthritis (adult)	Comments	Side effects
Naproxen (cont'd)	Oral	Napratec	Tablet	500mg (with misoprostol 200mcg)	1 of each tablet taken together 2 times/d	Used as prophylaxis against NSAID-induced gastroduodenal ulceration; contraindicated in pregnant women and women planning a pregnancy	
	Rectal	Naprosyn	Suppository	500mg	500-1000mg/d		Rectal irritation and occasional bleeding
Naproxen sodium	Oral	Anaprox	Tablet	375mg, 500mg	750-1000mg/d	Take with or after food	Gastrointestinal discomfort, nausea, diarrhoea; gastrointestinal bleeding and ulceration; hypersensitivity reactions; headache, dizziness, vertigo, hearing disturbances; renal papillary necrosis, renal decompensation in patients with renal impairment
Piroxicam	Oral	Feldene	Tablet; capsule	10mg, 20mg	10-30mg/d	Take with or after food	Gastrointestinal discomfort, nausea, diarrhoea; gastrointestinal bleeding and ulceration; hypersensitivity reactions; headache, dizziness, vertigo, hearing disturbances
	Topical	Feldene	Gel	0.5%	Apply 3-4 times/d		Hypersensitivity reactions
	Rectal	Feldene	Suppository	20mg	20mg/d		Rectal irritation and occasional bleeding
Sulindac	Oral	Clinoril	Tablet	100mg, 200mg	200mg 2 times/d	Take with or after food	Gastrointestinal discomfort, nausea, diarrhoea; gastrointestinal bleeding and ulceration; hypersensitivity reactions; headache, dizziness, vertigo, hearing disturbances
Tenoxicam	Oral	Mobiflex	Tablet	20mg	20mg/d	Take with or after food	Gastrointestinal discomfort, nausea, diarrhoea; gastrointestinal bleeding and ulceration; hypersensitivity reactions; headache, dizziness, vertigo, hearing disturbances
Tiaprofenic acid	Oral	Surgam	Tablet	200mg, 300mg	600mg/d in divided doses	Contraindicated in patients with urinary tract disorders as severe cystitis has been reported; take with or after food	Gastrointestinal discomfort, nausea, diarrhoea; gastrointestinal bleeding and ulceration; hypersensitivity reactions; headache, dizziness, vertigo, hearing disturbances
		Surgam SA	M/R capsule	300mg	600mg/d		

Cyclo-oxygenase 2 (Cox-2) inhibitors

Drug	Format	Trade name	Preparation	Strength	Doses used in arthritis (adult)	Comments	Side effects
Celecoxib	Oral	Celebrex	Capsule	100mg, 200mg	100-200mg 2 times/d	May be preferred to standard NSAIDs in patients with gastrointestinal ulceration or bleeding or in patients with a high risk of gastrointestinal adverse events; take with or after food	Gastrointestinal discomfort, flatulence, nausea, diarrhoea; gastrointestinal bleeding and ulceration; hypersensitivity reactions; insomnia, headache, dizziness, vertigo, hearing disturbances
Etoricoxib	Oral	Arcoxia	Tablet	60mg, 90mg, 120mg	OA 60mg/d; RA 90mg/d	May be preferred to standard NSAIDs in patients with gastrointestinal ulceration or bleeding or in patients with a high risk of gastrointestinal adverse events; contraindicated in severe congestive heart failure; take with or after food	Gastrointestinal discomfort, flatulence, dry mouth, taste disturbance, mouth ulcers, constipation, appetite and weight changes; gastrointestinal bleeding and ulceration; hypersensitivity reactions; fatigue, paraesthesia, myalgia, influenza type syndrome
Rofecoxib	Oral	Vioxx	Tablet	12.5mg, 25mg	12.5-25mg/d	May be preferred to standard NSAIDs in patients with gastrointestinal ulceration or bleeding or in patients with a high risk of gastrointestinal adverse events; take with or after food	Gastrointestinal discomfort, nausea, diarrhoea; gastrointestinal bleeding and ulceration; hypersensitivity reactions; sleep disturbance, headache, dizziness, vertigo, hearing disturbances, sweating, alopecia
Valdecoxib	Oral	Bextra	Tablet	10mg, 20mg, 40mg	10mg/d (max. 20mg/d)	May be preferred to standard NSAIDs in patients with gastrointestinal ulceration or bleeding or in patients with a high risk of gastrointestinal adverse events; contraindicated in severe congestive heart failure; take with or after food	Gastrointestinal discomfort, belching, dry mouth, taste disturbance, stomatitis, weight gain; gastrointestinal bleeding and ulceration; hypersensitivity reactions; palpitations, syncope, coughing, hypertonia, paraesthesia, confusion

Simple analgesia

Drug	Format	Trade name	Preparation	Strength	Doses used in arthritis (adult)	Comments	Side effects
Aspirin	Oral	Generic	Tablet	300mg	300-900mg 4-6h (max. 4000mg/d)	Take with or after food	Gastrointestinal discomfort, gastrointestinal bleeding and ulceration, increased bleeding time, nausea, hearing disturbances, bronchospasm, hypersensitivity reactions
		Caprin	E/C tablet	300mg			
		Nu-Seal	E/C tablet	300mg			
		Generic	Tablet	400mg (with codeine 8mg)	1-2 tablets 4-6h		
	Rectal	Generic	Suppository	300mg	600-900mg/4h		Rectal irritation and occasional bleeding
Benorylate	Oral	Benoral	Tablet	750mg	4000-8000mg/d in 2-3 divided doses; elderly max. 6g/d	Aspirin-paracetamol ester: 2g benorilate is equivalent to approximately 1.15g aspirin and 970mg paracetamol; take with or after food	Gastrointestinal discomfort, gastrointestinal bleeding and ulceration, increased bleeding time, nausea, hearing disturbances, bronchospasm, hypersensitivity reactions, rashes, blood disorders, acute pancreatitis
		Benoral	Granules	2000mg			
		Benoral	Suspension	5000mg/5ml			
Benzydamine	Topical	Difflam	Cream	3%	Apply 3-6 times/d		Hypersensitivity reactions
Capsaicin	Topical	Zacin	Cream	0.025%	Apply 4 times/d	Use sparingly	Transient burning sensation
Diethylamine salicylate	Topical	Algesal	Cream	10%	Apply 3 times/d		Hypersensitivity reactions
Ethyl nicotinate + hexyl nicotinate + thurfyl salicylate	Topical	Transvasin	Cream	2% + 2% + 14%	Apply 2 times/d		Hypersensitivity reactions
Heparinoid + salicylic acid + thymol	Topical	Movelat	Cream, gel	0.2% + 2% + 1%	Apply 4 times/d		Hypersensitivity reactions
Nefopam	Oral	Acupan	Tablet	30mg	60mg (elderly 30mg) 3 times/d (range 30-90mg 3 times/d)	Contraindicated in hepatic and renal disease, elderly, urinary retention; caution in pregnancy, breast feeding	Nausea, nervousness, urinary retention, dry mouth, light-headedness, vomiting, blurred vision, drowsiness, sweating, insomnia, tachycardia, headache

Simple analgesia

Drug	Format	Trade name	Preparation	Strength	Doses used in arthritis (adult)	Comments	Side effects
Paracetamol	Oral	Generic	Tablet	500mg	500-1000mg 3-4 times/d		Rashes, blood disorders, acute pancreatitis
		Generic	Suspension	250mg/5ml			
		Generic	Suppository	250mg	500-1000mg 2 times/d		
Paracetamol + codeine (co-codamol)	Oral	Generic	Tablet, capsule	500mg + 8mg	1-2 tablets or capsules 4 times/d		Rashes, blood disorders, acute pancreatitis, nausea, vomiting, constipation, drowsiness
		Codipar	Tablet	500mg + 15mg	1-2 capsules 4 times/d		
		Kapake, Solpadol, Tylex	Tablet, capsule	500mg + 30mg	1-2 tablets or capsules 4 times/d		
Paracetamol + dextro-propoxyphene (co-proxamol)	Oral	Generic	Tablet	325mg + 32.5mg	1-2 tablets 4 times/d	Special hazard in overdose and care in the elderly	Rashes, blood disorders, acute pancreatitis, nausea, vomiting, constipation, drowsiness, convulsions in overdose
		Distalgesic	Tablet	325mg + 32.5mg	1-2 tablets 4 times/d		
Paracetamol + dihydrocodeine (co-dydramol)	Oral	Generic	Tablet	500mg + 10mg	1-2 tablets 4 times/d		Rashes, blood disorders, acute pancreatitis, nausea, vomiting, constipation, drowsiness
		Remedene	Tablet	500mg + 20mg	1-2 tablets 4 times/d		
		Remedene Forte		500mg + 30mg	1-2 tablets 4 times/d		

Opioid analgesics

Drug	Format	Trade name	Preparation	Strength	Doses used in arthritis (adult)	Comments	Side effects
Buprenorphine	Oral	Tempgesic	Sublingual tablet	0.2mg, 0.4mg	0.2-0.4mg every 8h increasing to 0.2-0.4mg every 4-6h according to response	Contraindicated in acute respiratory depression; caution in hypotension, hypothyroidism, asthma, decreased respiratory reserve, pregnancy, breast feeding, hepatic and renal impairment, elderly; long acting opioid agonist/antagonist	Nausea, vomiting, constipation, drowsiness, difficulty with micturition, ureteric or biliary spasm, dry mouth, sweating, headache, facial flushing, vertigo, bradycardia, tachycardia, palpitations, postural hypotension, hypothermia, hallucinations, mood changes, dependence, rashes, urticaria, pruritus; mild withdrawal symptoms in patients dependent on opiates
	Transdermal	Transtec	Patch	35mcg/h, 52.5mcg/h, 70mcg/h	Apply 1 patch every 72h		
Codeine	Oral	Generic	Tablet	25mg, 30mg, 60mg	30-60mg every 4h (max. 240mg/d)	Contraindicated in acute respiratory depression; caution in hypotension, hypothyroidism, asthma, decreased respiratory reserve, pregnancy, breast feeding, hepatic and renal impairment, elderly	Nausea, vomiting, constipation, drowsiness, difficulty with micturition, ureteric or biliary spasm, dry mouth, sweating, headache, facial flushing, vertigo, bradycardia, tachycardia, palpitations, postural hypotension, hypothermia, hallucinations, mood changes, dependence, rashes, urticaria, pruritus
Dihydrocodeine	Oral	Generic	Tablet	30mg	30mg every 4-6h	Contraindicated in acute respiratory depression; caution in hypotension, hypothyroidism, asthma, decreased respiratory reserve, pregnancy, breast feeding, hepatic and renal impairment, elderly; M/R tablets should be swallowed whole	Nausea, vomiting, constipation, drowsiness, difficulty with micturition, ureteric or biliary spasm, dry mouth, sweating, headache, facial flushing, vertigo, bradycardia, tachycardia, palpitations, postural hypotension, hypothermia, hallucinations, mood changes, dependence, rashes, urticaria, pruritus
		DF 118 Forte	Tablet	40mg			
		DHC Continus	M/R tablet	60mg, 90mg, 120mg			
Fentanyl	Transdermal	Durogesic	Patch	25mcg/h, 50mcg/h, 75mcg/h, 100mcg/h	Apply 1 patch every 72h	Contraindicated in acute respiratory depression; caution in hypotension, hypothyroidism, asthma, decreased respiratory reserve, pregnancy, breast feeding, hepatic and renal impairment, elderly; long acting analgesia	Nausea, vomiting, constipation, drowsiness, difficulty with micturition, ureteric or biliary spasm, dry mouth, sweating, headache, facial flushing, vertigo, bradycardia, tachycardia, palpitations, postural hypotension, hypothermia, hallucinations, mood changes, dependence, rashes, urticaria, pruritus

Opioid analgesics

Drug	Format	Trade name	Preparation	Strength	Doses used in arthritis (adult)	Comments	Side effects
Meptazinol	Oral	Meptid	Tablet	200mg	200mg every 3-6h	Contraindicated in acute respiratory depression; caution in hypotension, hypothyroidism, asthma, decreased respiratory reserve, pregnancy, breast feeding, hepatic and renal impairment, elderly	Nausea, vomiting, constipation, drowsiness, difficulty with micturition, ureteric or biliary spasm, dry mouth, sweating, headache, facial flushing, vertigo, bradycardia, tachycardia, palpitations, postural hypotension, hypothermia, hallucinations, mood changes, dependence, rashes, urticaria, pruritus
Morphine		Morcap SR	M/R capsule	20mg, 50mg, 100mg	5-20mg every 4h, increasing according to response	Contraindicated in acute respiratory depression; caution in hypotension, hypothyroidism, asthma, decreased respiratory reserve, pregnancy, breast feeding, hepatic and renal impairment, elderly; M/R capsules should be swallowed whole or opened and sprinkled on soft food	Nausea, vomiting, constipation, drowsiness, respiratory depression and hypotension (large doses); difficulty with micturition, ureteric or biliary spasm, dry mouth, sweating, headache, facial flushing, vertigo, bradycardia, tachycardia, palpitations, postural hypotension, hypothermia, hallucinations, mood changes, dependence, rashes, urticaria, pruritus
		MST Continus	M/R tablet	5mg, 10mg, 15mg, 30mg, 60mg, 100mg, 200mg			
		MXL	M/R capsule	30mg, 60mg, 90mg,120mg, 150mg, 200mg			
		Oramorph	Oral solution	10mg/5ml			
				100mg/5ml			
		Sevredol	Oral solution	10mg/5ml			
				100mg/5ml			
			Tablet	10mg, 20mg, 50mg			
		Zomorph	M/R capsule	10mg, 30mg, 60mg, 100mg, 200mg			

Opioid analgesics

Drug	Format	Trade name	Preparation	Strength	Doses used in arthritis (adult)	Comments	Side effects
Pentazocine	Oral	Generic	Tablet	25mg	50mg every 3–4h (range 25–100mg; max. 600mg/d)	Contraindicated in acute respiratory depression, porphyria, hypertension, heart failure; caution in hypotension, hypothyroidism, asthma, decreased respiratory reserve, pregnancy, breast feeding, hepatic and renal impairment, elderly	Nausea, vomiting, constipation, drowsiness, difficulty with micturition, ureteric or biliary spasm, dry mouth, sweating, headache, facial flushing, vertigo, bradycardia, tachycardia, palpitations, postural hypotension, hypothermia, hallucinations, mood changes, dependence, rashes, urticaria, pruritus
			Capsule	50mg			
Pethidine	Oral	Generic	Tablet	50mg	50–100mg every 4h	Contraindicated in acute respiratory depression; caution in hypotension, hypothyroidism, asthma, decreased respiratory reserve, pregnancy, breast feeding, hepatic and renal impairment, elderly; do not use in severe, continuing pain	Nausea, vomiting, constipation, drowsiness, difficulty with micturition, ureteric or biliary spasm, dry mouth, sweating, headache, facial flushing, vertigo, bradycardia, tachycardia, palpitations, postural hypotension, hypothermia, hallucinations, mood changes, dependence, rashes, urticaria, pruritus
Tramadol	Oral	Generic	Capsule	50mg	50–100mg every 4h increasing according to response; SR preparations 50–200mg 2 times/d; XL preparations 150mg/d increasing according to response (max. 400mg/d) for all preparations	Contraindicated in acute respiratory depression, pregnancy, breast feeding; caution in epilepsy, hypotension, hypothyroidism, asthma, decreased respiratory reserve; caution in hepatic and renal impairment, elderly; M/R preparations should be swallowed whole	Nausea, vomiting, constipation, drowsiness, difficulty with micturition, ureteric or biliary spasm, dry mouth, sweating, headache, facial flushing, vertigo, bradycardia, tachycardia, palpitations, postural hypotension, hypothermia, hallucinations, mood changes, dependence, rashes, urticaria, pruritus
		Zamadol, Zydol	Capsule	50mg			
		Dromadol SR	M/R tablet (2 times/d dosing)	75mg, 100mg, 150mg, 200mg			
		Dromadol XL; Zydol XL	M/R tablet (once daily dosing)	150mg, 200mg, 300mg, 400mg			
		Zamadol SR	M/R capsule (2 times/d dosing)	50mg, 100mg, 150mg, 200mg			
		Zydol SR	M/R tablet (once daily dosing)	100mg, 150mg, 200mg			

Corticosteroids

Drug	Format	Trade name	Preparation	Strength	Doses used in arthritis (adult)	Comments	Side effects
Dexamethasone sodium phosphate	Parenteral	Generic	Intra-articular or intrasynovial injection	4.4mg/ml, 5mg/ml	0.4-4mg by intra-articular or intrasynovial injection every 3-21 days	See prednisolone	See prednisolone
Hydrocortisone acetate	Parenteral	Hydro-cortistab	Intra-articular or intrasynovial injection	25mg/ml	5-50mg by intra-articular or intrasynovial injection (max. 3 joints/d) every 21 days	See prednisolone	See prednisolone
Methyl-prednisolone acetate	Parenteral	Depo-Medrone	Intra-articular or intrasynovial injection	40mg/ml	4-80mg by intra-articular or intrasynovial injection every 7-35 days	See prednisolone	See prednisolone
		Depo-Medrone with Lidocaine	Intra-articular or intrasynovial injection	40mg/ml (+ lidocaine 10mg/ml)			
Prednisolone	Oral	Generic	Tablet	1mg, 5mg	Initial dose usually 10-20mg/d (max. 60mg); maintenance 2.5-15mg/d	Contraindicated in systemic infection; caution in adrenal suppression, adolescents, elderly, hypertension, recent myocardial infarction, congestive heart failure, hepatic and renal impairment, diabetes mellitus, osteoporosis, glaucoma, severe affective disorders, epilepsy, peptic ulcer, hypothyroidism, pregnancy, breast feeding; oral dose preferably taken each morning after breakfast	Gastrointestinal effects (dyspepsia, peptic ulceration, abdominal distension, acute pancreatitis, oesophageal ulceration, candidiasis); musculoskeletal effects (osteoporosis, vertebral and long bone fractures, tendon rupture); endocrine effects (adrenal suppression, menstrual abnormalities and amenorrhoea, Cushing's syndrome, hirsutism, weight gain); neuropsychiatric effects (euphoria, psychological dependence, depression, insomnia, psychosis); ophthalmic effects (glaucoma, cataract, corneal thinning); impaired healing, skin atrophy, bruising, acne, fluid and electrolyte disturbances; injection - injection site reactions, local necrosis and muscle wasting, Charcot-like arthropathy, effects on hyaline cartridge
		Deltacortril	E/C tablet	2.5mg, 5mg			
		Precortisyl Forte	Tablet	25mg			
	Parenteral	Deltastab	Intra-articular or intrasynovial injection	25mg/ml	5-25mg by intra-articular or intrasynovial injection (max. 3 joints/d)		
Triamcinolone acetonide	Parenteral	Kenalog	Intra-articular or intrasynovial injection	10mg/ml, 40mg/ml	2.5-40mg by intra-articular or intrasynovial injection (max. 80mg)	See prednisolone	See prednisolone

Hyaluronans

Drug	Format	Trade name	Preparation	Strength	Doses used in arthritis (adult)	Comments	Side effects
Hyaluronic acid (synthetic)	Parenteral	Durolane	Intra-articular injection	20mg/ml	3ml as a single intra-articular injection, repeat after 6m prn	Used for mild to moderate OA of the knee, remove joint effusion prior to injection; contraindicated in infection or skin disease at injection site, infection or severe inflammation of the knee; caution in venous or lymphatic stasis, pregnancy, breast feeding	Pain and swelling at injection site
Hyaluronic acid (sodium salt, avian)	Parenteral	Hyalgan	Intra-articular injection	20mg/2ml	2ml by intra-articular injection once weekly for a total of 5 injections; repeat course at 6m intervals prn	Used to provide sustained relief of pain in OA of the knee, remove joint effusion prior to injection; contraindicated in hypersensitivity to avian proteins, infection or skin disease at injection site, caution in acute joint inflammation, pregnancy, breast feeding	Transient pain, swelling and heat at injection site
Hylan G-F 20 (avian)	Parenteral	Synvisc	Intra-articular injection	8mg/ml	Knee: 2ml by intra-articular weekly for 3w, repeat prn with min. 4w between courses (max. 6 injections in 6m); hip: 2ml as a single intra-articular injection, repeat prn after 1-3m	Used in OA of hip and knee; contraindicated in hypersensitivity to avian proteins, venous or lymphatic stasis of the leg, infected or severely inflamed joints, caution in pregnancy, breast feeding	Transient pain and swelling at injection site
Sodium hyaluronate (synthetic)	Parenteral	Ostenil	Intra-articular injection	20mg/2ml	2ml by intra-articular injection once weekly for up to 5 injections; repeat course at 6m intervals prn	Used to improve pain and restricted mobility in degenerative and traumatic changes of the knee and other synovial joints, remove joint effusion prior to injection; contraindicated in infection or skin disease at injection site; caution in pregnancy, breast feeding	Pain and swelling at injection site

Disease modifying antirheumatic drugs (DMARDs)

Drug	Format	Trade name	Preparation	Strength	Doses used in arthritis (adult)	Comments	Side effects
Auranofin	Oral	Ridaura	Tablet	3mg	Expert advice: 3mg 2 times/d increasing to 3mg 3 times/d after 6 months if response is inadequate	Used for active progressive RA; contraindicated in severe renal and hepatic disease, history of blood or bone marrow disorders, exfoliative dermatitis, systemic lupus erythematosus, necrotizing enterocolitis, pulmonary fibrosis, pregnancy, breastfeeding; caution in elderly, history of urticaria, eczema, inflammatory bowel disease; take with or after food	Severe hypersensitivity reactions, mouth ulcers, skin reactions, diarrhoea, irreversible pigmentation in sun exposed areas following prolonged treatment, proteinuria, blood disorders (sometimes sudden and fatal), colitis, peripheral neuritis, pulmonary fibrosis, hepatotoxicity, nephrotic syndrome, alopecia; take with or after food
Azathioprine	Oral	Generic	Tablet	25mg, 50mg	Expert advice: 1.5-2.5mg/kg/d in divided doses (maintenance 1-3mg/kg/d)	Used for moderate to severe RA which has not responded to other DMARDs; caution in renal and hepatic impairment, pregnancy, elderly (reduce dose)	Hypersensitivity reactions (malaise, dizziness, vomiting, diarrhoea, fever, rigors, myalgia, arthralgia, disturbed liver function, rash, hypotension, interstitial nephritis), bone marrow suppression, hair loss and increased susceptibility to infections and colitis in patients also receiving corticosteroids, nausea
		Imuran	Tablet	25mg, 50mg			
Chloroquine	Oral	Avloclor	Tablet	150mg (base)	Expert advice: 150mg base/d	Used for active RA; contraindicated in breast-feeding; caution in hepatic and renal impairment, neurological disorders (especially epilepsy), severe gastrointestinal disorders, G6PD deficiency, porphyria, elderly, pregnancy	Exacerbation of psoriasis and aggravation of myasthenia gravis; gastrointestinal disturbances, headache, skin reactions (rashes, pruritus), ECG changes, convulsions, visual changes, retinal damage, keratopathy, ototoxicity, hair depigmentation, alopecia, discolouration of skin, nails and mucous membranes
		Nivaquine	Tablet	150mg (base)			
			Syrup	50mg (base)/5ml			
Cyclosporine	Oral	Neoral	Capsule	10mg, 25mg, 50mg, 100mg	Expert advice: 1.25mg/kg 2 times/d (max. 4mg/kg/d)	Used for severe active RA when conventional second line therapy is ineffective; contraindicated in uncontrolled hypertension, uncontrolled infections, malignancy; caution in pregnancy, breastfeeding	Disturbances in renal function (increased serum creatinine and urea), renal structural changes (long-term administration), hypertrichosis, tremor, hypertension, hepatic dysfunction, fatigue, gingival hypertrophy, gastrointestinal disturbances, burning sensation in hands and feet
			Oral solution	100mg/ml			

Disease modifying antirheumatic drugs (DMARDs)

Drug	Format	Trade name	Preparation	Strength	Doses used in arthritis (adult)	Comments	Side effects
Cyclophosphamide	Oral	Generic	Tablet	50mg	Expert advice: 1-1.5mg/kg/d orally or 0.5-1g by IV injection with prophylactic mensa every 2-4 weeks	Used for RA with severe systemic manifestations; contraindicated in pregnancy, breastfeeding, porphyria; caution in hepatic and renal impairment	Gastrointestinal disturbances, haematological disturbances, haemorrhagic cystitis (ensure adequate hydration)
	Parenteral	Generic	IV injection	200mg			
	Oral	Endoxana	Tablet	50mg			
	Parenteral	Endoxana	IV injection	200mg			
Hydroxychloroquine	Oral	Plaquenil	Tablet	200mg	Expert advice: 200mg 2 times/d (maintenance 200-400mg/d)	Used for active RA; contraindicated in breast-feeding; caution in hepatic and renal impairment, neurological disorders (especially epilepsy), severe gastrointestinal disorders, G6PD deficiency, porphyria, elderly, pregnancy; take with or after food	Exacerbation of psoriasis and aggravation of myasthenia gravis; gastrointestinal disturbances, headache, skin reactions (rashes, pruritus), ECG changes, convulsions, visual changes, retinal damage, keratopathy, ototoxicity, hair depigmentation, alopecia, discolouration of skin, nails and mucous membranes
Leflunomide	Oral	Arava	Tablet	10mg, 20mg, 100mg	Expert advice: 100mg/d for 3 days (maintenance 10-20mg/d)	Used for moderate to severe RA when sulfasalazine or methotrexate cannot be used; contraindicated in severe immunodeficiency, serious infection, hepatic impairment, severe hypoproteinaemia, pregnancy (teratogenic), breastfeeding; caution in renal impairment, impaired bone marrow function	Diarrhoea, nausea, vomiting, anorexia, oral mucosal disorders, abdominal pain, weight loss, hypertension, headache, dizziness, asthenia, paraesthesia, tenosynovitis, alopecia, eczema, dry skin, rash, pruritus, leucopenia; teratogenic - effective contraception essential during treatment and for > 2 years after treatment (women) and > 3 months after treatment (men)
Methotrexate	Oral	Generic	Tablet	2.5mg, 10mg	Expert advice: 7.5mg/week (max. 20mg/week)	Used for moderate to severe RA; contraindicated in severe hepatic and renal impairment, active infection, immunodeficiency syndromes, breastfeeding; caution in blood disorders, peptic ulceration, ulcerative colitis, diarrhoea, ulcerative stomatitis, photosensitivity, porphyria	Gastrointestinal disturbances, myelosuppression, haematological disturbances, pulmonary toxicity, teratogenic - effective contraception essential during treatment and for 3 months after treatment (men and women)
		Maxtrex	Tablet	2.5mg, 10mg			

Disease modifying antirheumatic drugs (DMARDs)

Drug	Format	Trade name	Preparation	Strength	Doses used in arthritis (adult)	Comments	Side effects
Penicillamine	Oral	Generic	Tablet	125mg, 250mg	Expert advice: 125-250mg/d increasing to maintenance 500-750mg/d in divided doses (max. 1.5g/d, elderly 1g/d)	Used for severe active RA; contraindicated in hypersensitivity, lupus erythematosus; caution in renal impairment, pregnancy; take before food	Nausea, anorexia, fever, skin reactions, taste loss, blood disorders (thrombocytopenia, neutropenia, agranulocytosis, aplastic anaemia), haematuria
		Distamine	Tablet	125mg, 250mg			
Sodium aurothiomalate	Parenteral	Myocrisin	I/M injection	20mg/ml, 40mg/ml, 100mg/ml	Expert advice: 10mg test dose; 50mg/week until response seen (6-8 weeks) then reduce frequency to maintain remission	Used for active progressive rheumatoid arthritis; contraindicated in severe renal and hepatic disease, history of blood or bone marrow disorders, exfoliative dermatitis, systemic lupus erythematosus, necrotizing enterocolitis, pulmonary fibrosis, pregnancy, breastfeeding; caution in elderly, history of urticaria, eczema, colitis	Severe hypersensitivity reactions in up to 5% of patients, mouth ulcers, skin reactions, irreversible pigmentation in sun exposed areas following prolonged treatment, proteinuria, blood disorders (sometimes sudden and fatal), colitis, peripheral neuritis, pulmonary fibrosis, hepatotoxicity, nephrotic syndrome, alopecia
Sulfasalazine (sulphasalazine)	Oral	Generic	Tablet	500mg	Expert advice: 500mg/d (max. 2-3g/d in divided doses)	Used for active RA; contraindicated in salicylate hypersensitivity, moderate or severe renal impairment; caution in pregnancy, breastfeeding	Nausea, vomiting, headache, loss of appetite, fever, haematological abnormalities (leucopenia, neutropenia, thrombocytopenia), hypersensitivity reactions, pulmonary toxicity (eosinophilia, fibrosing alveolitis), ocular complications, stomatitis, parotitis, ataxia, aseptic meningitis, vertigo, tinnitus, peripheral neuropathy, insomnia, depression, hallucinations
		Salazopyrin	Tablet	500mg			
			E/C tablet	500mg			

169

Biological agents affecting the immune response

Drug	Format	Trade name	Preparation	Strength	Doses used in arthritis (adult)	Comments	Side effects
Adalimumab	Parenteral	Humira	S/C injection	40mg	Expert advice: 40mg every 2 weeks (max 40mg/ week in patients not taking methotrexate)	Used for moderate to severe active RA which has not responded to at least 1 standard DMARD; contraindicated in immuno-suppressed patients, patients with active or chronic infection; caution in patients with conditions that predispose them to infections (e.g. diabetes), CNS demyelinating disorders, haematological disorders, cardiac disease, elderly, pregnancy, breastfeeding	Increased incidence of serious infections (including pneumonia, septic arthritis, prosthetic and post-surgical infections, erysipelas, cellulitis, diverticulitis, pyelonephritis), injection site reactions (erythema, inflammation, pain), haematological abnormalities (agranulocytosis, granulocytopenia, leukopenia, lymphoma), hypersensitivity reactions (asthma, bronchospasm, rash), headache, nausea, abdominal pain, sinusitis
Anakinra	Parenteral	Kineret	S/C injection	100mg	Expert advice: 100mg/d	Used for highly active progressive RA which has not responded to at least 2 standard DMARDs including methotrexate; contraindicated in immunosuppressed patients, patients with active or chronic infections; caution in asthma, severe renal impairment, elderly, pregnancy, breastfeeding	Increased incidence of serious infections (mainly cellulitis, pneumonia, bone and joint infections - risk further increased when given with concurrent etanercept or infliximab), injection site reactions (erythema, inflammation, pain), haematological effects (neutropenia), hypersensitivity reactions, headache, nausea, diarrhoea, sinusitis
Etanercept	Parenteral	Enbrel	S/C injection	25mg	Expert advice: 25mg 2 times/ week	Used for highly active progressive RA which has not responded to at least 2 standard DMARDs; contraindicated in patients with active or chronic infections; caution in patients with conditions that predispose them to infections (e.g. diabetes), CNS demyelinating disorders, worsening heart failure, elderly, pregnancy, breastfeeding	Increased incidence of serious infections (mainly upper respiratory tract infections, also pyelonephritis, bronchitis, abdominal abscess, cellulitis, osteomyelitis, would infection, pneumonia, foot abscess, leg ulcers, sepsis - risk further increased when given with concurrent anakinra), injection site reactions (erythema, itching, pain, swelling), haematological effects (pancytopenia), transverse myelitis, optic neuritis, multiple sclerosis, new onset or exacerbation of seizure disorders, hypersensitivity reactions, headache, nausea, diarrhoea, sinusitis

Biological agents affecting the immune response

Drug	Format	Trade name	Preparation	Strength	Doses used in arthritis (adult)	Comments	Side effects
Infliximab	Parenteral	Remicade	IV injection (for infusion)	100mg	Expert advice: 3mg/kg by IV infusion, repeated after 2 and 6 weeks and then every 8 weeks (max. 10mg/kg)	Used for highly active progressive RA which has not responded to at least 2 standard DMARDs including methotrexate; contraindicated in patients with active or chronic infections, severe congestive heart failure; caution in immunosuppressed patients, patients with CNS demyelinating disorders, mild or moderate congestive heart failure, elderly, pregnancy, breastfeeding	Increased incidence of serious infections (mainly respiratory tract and urinary tract infections – risk further increased when given with concurrent anakinra), disseminated or extrapulmonary tuberculosis, infusion related reactions (fever, chills, chest pain, hypotension, hypertension, dyspnoea, pruritus, urticaria at injection site), haematological effects,worsening heart failure, optic neuritis, multiple sclerosis, new onset or exacerbation of seizure disorders, hypersensitivity reactions, headache, sinusitis

Abbreviations

ACL	Anterior cruciate ligament
ACR	American College of Rheumatology
ANA	Anti-nuclear antibody
arc	Arthritis Research Campaign
BNF	British National Formulary
CCP	Cyclic, citrullinated peptides
CMC	Carpometacarpal
CNS	Central nervous system
Cox-2s	Cyclo-oxygenase 2 inhibitors
CRP	C-reactive protein
CT	Computed tomography
CTD	Connective tissue disease
CWP	Chronic widespread pain
DAS	Disease Activity Score
DEXA	Dual-energy X-ray absorptiometry
DIP	Distal interphalangeal
DMARD	Disease-modifying anti-rheumatic drug
DOH	Department of Health
ENA	Extractable nuclear antigens
ESR	Erythrocyte sedimentation rate
ESWT	Extracorporeal shock wave therapy
GCA	Giant cell arteritis
GP	General Practitioner
GPwSI	General Practitioner with a special interest
HIV	Human immunodeficiency virus
HLA	Human leukocyte antigen
Ig	Immunoglobulin
IL	Interleukin
IP	Interphalangeal
MCP	Metacarpophalangeal
MRI	Magnetic resonance imaging
MSK	Musculoskeletal medicine
MTP	Metatarsophalangeal
NHS	National Health Service
NICE	National Institute for Clinical Excellence
NIH	US National Institutes of Health
NNT	Number needed to treat
NO	Nitric oxide
NRAS	National RA Society
NSAID	Non-steroidal anti-inflammatory drug
OA	Osteoarthritis
OT	Occupational therapy
OTC	Over the counter
PCT	Primary Care Trust
PIP	Proximal interphalangeal
PMR	Polymyalgia rheumatica
RA	Rheumatoid arthritis
RCT	Randomized controlled trial
RF	Rheumatoid factor
RP	Raynaud's phenomenon
RSD	Reflex sympathetic dystrophy
RSI	Repetitive strain injury
SjS	Sjögren's syndrome
SLE	Systemic lupus erythematosus
TB	Tuberculosis
TENS	Transcutaneous electrical nerve stimulation
TNF	Tumour necrosis factor
WHO	World Health Organization
WOMAC	Western Ontario and McMaster
WRULD	Work-related upper limb disorder

Arc 1987 Criteria for the Classification of Acute Arthritis of Rheumatoid Arthritis

A patient has rheumatoid arthritis if he/she has satisfied at least 4 of these 7 criteria.
The first 4 criteria must have been present for at least 6 weeks.
Patients with 2 clinical diagnoses are not excluded.

Criterion	Definition
Morning stiffness	Morning stiffness in and around the joints, lasting ≥ 1 hour before maximal improvement
Arthritis of ≥ 3 joint areas	≥ 3 joint areas simultaneously have had soft tissue swelling or fluid (not bony overgrowth alone) observed by a physician. The 14 possible areas are right or left PIP, MCP, wrist, elbow, knee, ankle, and MTP joints
Arthritis of hand joints	≥ 1 area swollen (as defined above) in a wrist, MCP, or PIP joint
Symmetric arthritis	Simultaneous involvement of the same joint areas (defined above) on both sides of the body (bilateral involvement of PIPs, MCPs or MTPs is acceptable without absolute symmetry)
Rheumatoid nodules	Subcutaneous nodules, over bony prominences, or extensor surfaces, or in juxta-articular regions, observed by a physician
Serum rheumatoid factor	Demonstration of abnormal amounts of serum RF by any method for which the result has been positive in < 5% of normal control subjects
Radiographic changes	Radiographic changes typical of RA on posteroanterior hand and wrist radiographs, which must include erosions or unequivocal bony decalcification localized in or most marked adjacent to the involved joints (OA changes alone do not qualify)

1982 Revised Criteria for Classification of Systemic Lupus Erythematosus

A person has SLE if any 4 or more of the 11 criteria are present, serially or simultaneously, during any interval of observation.

Criterion	Definition
Malar rash	Fixed erythema, flat or raised, over the malar eminences, tending to spare the nasolabial folds
Discoid rash	Erythematous raised patches with adherent keratotic scaling and follicular plugging; atrophic scarring may occur in older lesions
Photosensitivity	Skin rash as a result of unusual reaction to sunlight, by patient history or physician observation
Oral ulcers	Oral or nasopharyngeal ulceration, usually painless, observed by physician
Arthritis	Nonerosive arthritis involving ≥ 2 peripheral joints, characterized by tenderness, swelling, or effusion
Serositis	a) Pleuritis: convincing history of pleuritic pain or rubbing heard by a physician or evidence of pleural effusion OR b) Pericarditis: documented by ECG or rub or evidence of pericardial effusion
Renal disorder	a) Persistent proteinuria > 0.5g/day, or > 3+ if quantitation not performed OR b) Cellular casts: may be red cell, haemoglobin, granular, tubular, or mixed
Neurologic disorder	a) Seizures: in the absence of offending drugs or known metabolic derangements; e.g., uraemia, ketoacidosis, or electrolyte imbalance OR b) Psychosis: in the absence of offending drugs or known metabolic derangements, e.g., uraemia, ketoacidosis, or electrolyte imbalance
Haematologic disorder	a) Haemolytic anaemia: with reticulocytosis OR b) Leukopenia: $< 4000/mm^3$ total on ≥ 2 occasions OR c) Lymphopenia: $< 1500/mm^3$ on ≥ 2 occasions OR d) Thrombocytopenia: $< 100,000/mm^3$ in the absence of offending drugs
Immunologic disorder	a) Positive LE cell preparation OR b) Anti-DNA: antibody to native DNA in abnormal titre OR c) Anti-Sm: presence of antibody to Sm nuclear antigen OR d) False positive serologic test for syphilis known to be positive for ≥ 6 months and confirmed by *Treponema pallidum* immobilization or fluorescent treponemal antibody absorption test
Antinuclear antibody	An abnormal titre of antinuclear antibody by immunofluorescence or an equivalent assay at any point in time and in the absence of drugs known to be associated with "drug-induced lupus" syndrome

1990 Diagnostic Criteria for Giant Cell (Temporal) Arteritis	
A patient has giant cell (temporal) arteritis if ≥ 3 of these 5 criteria are present.	
Criterion	**Definition**
Age at disease onset ≥ 50 years	Development of symptoms or findings beginning at ≥ 50 years
New headache	New onset of or new type of localized pain in the head
Temporal artery abnormality	Temporal artery tenderness to palpation or decreased pulsation, unrelatd to arteriosclerosis of cervical arteries
Elevated ESR	ESR ≥ 50mm/hour by the Westergren method
Abnormal artery biopsy	Biopsy specimen with artery showing vasculitis characterized by a predominance of mononuclear cell infiltration or granulomatous inflammation, usually with multinucleated giant cells

Guidelines

PCR guidelines

The Primary Care Rheumatology Society have developed various guidelines, which are available at http://www.pcrsociety.org.uk or from The Primary Care Rheumatology Society, PO Box 42, Northallerton, North Yorkshire, DL7 8YG (Tel: +44 (0)1609 774794). These include guidelines on the management of knee OA (Fig. 72) and minimum standard guidelines for osteoporosis (Fig. 73).

RCP guideline

The Royal College of Physicians has prepared a concise guide to the prevention and treatment of glucocorticoid-induced osteoporosis (see summary guidance page 180).

Glucocorticoid-induced osteoporosis: A concise guide to prevention and treatment

This guide summarises evidence-based guidelines for the management of glucocorticoid-induced osteoporosis[1] developed by the Bone and Tooth Society of Great Britain, the National Osteoporosis Society and the Royal College of Physicians. Since 1997 several important epidemiological and intervention studies have been published which provide a substantial increase in the available data on glucocorticoid-induced osteoporosis. These guidelines are timely because they complement the Royal College of Physicians *Guidelines on the prevention and treatment of osteoporosis*[2,3] and the recent *National service framework for older people*[4] in which the problem of osteoporosis is emphasised in the section on falls. In addition, in 1998 the National Osteoporosis Society issued a guidance document on the management of glucocorticoid-induced osteoporosis.[5]

The need for evidence-based guidelines on the management of osteoporosis was recognised by the Department of Health Advisory Group on Osteoporosis in 1994. Following the publication of the NHS White Papers, *The new NHS: modern, dependable*[6] and *Saving lives: our healthier nation*,[7] and with the establishment of the National Institute for Clinical Excellence, there has been further emphasis on systematically generated evidence on which clinical management can be based.

Epidemiological data suggest that the current population at risk of developing glucocorticoid-induced fractures in the United Kingdom might be as large as 350,000, and that the vast majority of glucocorticoid-treated individuals have not been evaluated for osteoporosis risk, or commenced on treatment to prevent bone loss and reduce the risk of fracture. In writing these guidelines, evidence-based methodology has been followed, with stratification of evidence to provide an up-to-

Fig. 72 Guidelines on the management of knee OA. Reprinted from the Primary Care Rheumatology Society. (opposite page)

KNEE OSTEOARTHRITIS
MANAGEMENT OPTIONS

Typical features of osteoarthritis

- Pain, especially use-related pain (worse on stairs and hills if patellofemoral OA)
- Pain affecting one or a few regions only (often bilateral signs)
- Stiffness after inactivity ('gelling') and in early morning (<30 minutes)
- Joint line and/or periarticular tenderness
- Reduced joint movement and function

- Bony swelling
- Coarse crepitus
- Only mild to modest effusion (if at all)
- Popliteal cyst
- Muscle wasting
- Age >=45 (F>M)
- May have Heberden's and/or Bouchard's nodes (especially women)

Suggested order of drug treatments – can be used in combination

- Paracetamol ⟶ • Topical NSAIDs ⟶ • Topical capsaicin ⟶ • Compound analgesics ⟶
- Oral NSAIDs ⟶ • Steroid injection ⟶ • Intra-articular hyaluronan injection

Management objectives – Essentials for every patient   Δ Education   + Pain relief   * Optimise function   ^ Modify structural progression

- Education (nature of OA, good prognosis, many treatment options, self-management) +Δ*
- Lifestyle modification
- Weight loss and dietary advice, if obese Δ*^
- Exercise: quadriceps strengthening, general (aerobic) fitness +*

- Footwear: 4 essential qualities
  1. flat
  2. thick/soft sole (preferably air-filled)
  3. broad forefoot
  4. soft upper (many good training shoes satisfy these requirements) +*
- Pacing activities: break up activity throughout the day, prioritise essential activities +*
- Simple, safe, effective analgesia: paracetamol (up to 1g four times daily)

Further Options

- Local heat or cold: ice pack, hot water bottle, heat lamp, OTC rubs +
- Topical NSAIDs: safe, often effective, patient-controlled, can be bought OTC +
- Topical capsaicin: often effective, beware eye contact +
- Physiotherapy: education, pain relief, exercise instruction, patella taping, TENS, walking aids: including sticks Δ+*
- Intra-articular steroid injection: no predictors of response; quick pain relief (1-2 days); may last 2-6 weeks; considered safe up to 4 times per year for inflammatory flares +
- Course of intra-articular hyaluronan injections (weekly for 3-5 weeks); as effective as steroid; delayed pain relief (1-3 weeks); may last several months +
- Drug options: other analgesics (compound/combined opiates), oral NSAIDs, low dose amitriptyline for chronic pain (especially with non-restorative sleep) +

Red Flags

- Fever/systemically unwell (? sepsis)
- Marked effusion, warmth, erythema (? sepsis, gout, pseudogout, haemarthrosis, HIV infection). Consider immediate referral to hospital
- Progressive, severe pain, predominantly at night (? malignancy, avascular necrosis)

Pointers to other diagnoses

- Age <45
- Referred pain (back, hip) in presence of normal knee examination
- History of locking and/or giving way (? meniscal tear, osteochondral bodies)
- Discrete swelling away from the joint (? pre-patellar bursitis)
- Multiple regional pain (? fibromyalgia, polyarthritis/rheumatoid arthritis)
- Marked inflammation: severe early morning stiffness, large tense effusion (? inflammatory arthritis, rheumatoid arthritis, pseudogout, gout, reactive arthritis, psoriatic arthritis)
- Sepsis

Reasons for referral

- Diagnostic uncertainty
- Persistent, poorly controlled pain
- Difficult management (local locking, pseudogout, drug side effects)
- Facilities not available locally, e.g. physiotherapy
- Multiple regional pain (? fibromyalgia, polyarthritis/rheumatoid arthritis)
- Surgery (persistent/severe pain, marked functional impairment, progressive deformity)
- Patient request for further reassurance

Full guideline available from: The Primary Care Rheumatology Society, PO Box 42, Northallerton, North Yorkshire. DL7 8YG

OSTEOPOROSIS: MINIMUM STANDARD GUIDELINES

Which patients should be treated?

The following patients should either be currently on treatment, or have it documented that they have been offered it:

- Corticosteroid users
- Early menopause
- Previous osteoporotic fracture

Treatment

Commence treatment for osteoporosis with one of the following:

- HRT • Biphosphonates • Calcitriol

Definitions	
Corticosteroid	Oral prednisolone >7.5mg if likely to be on this for >3 months and >50 years old (or >15mg if <50 years old)
Early menopause	Cessation of ovarian function at 45 years old
Osteoporotic fracture	Fractures sustained from a fall while patient is standing on ground, especially if >60 years old, or wedge fracture of spine without major trauma

For patients over 60 years of age	Any of these treatments can be used as a first choice: the first choice depends on the patient. Factors to be considered include:
	• likelihood of patient compliance
	• acceptability of side-effect profile to patient
	• ease of medication regimen
Early menopause	HRT should be advised
Corticosteroid users	The first choice treatment depends on whether the patient is pre- or post-menopausal

Other Information

The elderly

- Dietary deficiency of calcium and vitamin D is very common
- As a general measure consider putting nursing home elderly on calcium and vitamin D tablets
- The management of osteoporosis is the same although the first choice of drugs may be more influenced by compliance issues
- Assess osteoporosis risk in daughters of any identified case
- The patient's perception of loss of height is usually correct (height measurement is not informative)

Selective oestrogen receptor modulators (SERMs)

- Oestrogen receptors are found in the following locations:
  - breast
  - uterus
  - cardiovascular system
  - bone
- Drugs have been developed that have a positive effect on bone and CVS, a neutral effect on uterus and may have a protective effect on breasts

General Advice

- If in doubt ask your local specialist

AREA FOR LABEL NAME AND CONTACT DETAILS OF LOCAL SPECIALIST

Patient information

Make the following points to the patient (they can be put on paper for the patient to take away):

- osteoporosis means thin bones that break more easily
- it is not painful except when a bone is broken or a vertebra is compressed
- it is very common, especially in women
- often there is no particular cause
- the only way it could affect you is if you broke a bone because it got thin
- we can stop bones getting thinner with treatment
- following your treatment regularly will stop this from happening
- information leaflets are available from your doctor or practice nurse

Investigations

- >90% of women will have no secondary cause
- Investigation should not delay treatment
- Investigations you might consider in relevant patients if secondary causes are suspected:
  - FSH: detect menopause in hysterectomised women with ovaries conserved
  - FBC: malabsorption
  - viscosity or ESR: multiple myeloma
  - electrolytes and urea: renal disease
  - LFT: chronic liver disease
  - TFT: occult hyperthyroidism or excess replacement in hypothyroidism
  - calcium: hyperparathyroidism
  - testosterone: hypogonadism in men
- <=50% of males have secondary causes, specialist referral may be appropriate

Other cases
Once the main at risk groups have been treated, the other groups at high risk can be sought

Risk factors include:	DXA scanning

Remember: osteoporosis may occur in those without risk factors
 	
- family history
- alcohol excess
- hyperthyroidism
- hyperparathyroidism
- maternal hip fracture
- anorexia
- amenorrhoea (>6 months)
- malabsorption
- smoking
 	
Patients may be considered for treatment if they have multiple risks. They can be considered for DXA scan if available
	Only use if result will change management
	• DXA not necessary in:
	  - women willing to take HRT
	  - elderly or frail
	• DXA may be useful in:
	  - women reluctant to take long-term therapy
	  - patients with risk factors outside the three main groups
	  - monitoring response to therapy as <=20% may not respond
	If DXA not available or long delay, do not delay treatment: commence therapy and scan when available

Full guideline available from:

The Primary Care Rheumatology Society, PO Box 42, Northallerton, North Yorkshire. DL7 8YG

Primary Care Rheumatology Society, Osteoporosis: minimum standard guidelines for PCR members. February 1999

Fig. 73 Minimum standard guidelines for osteoporosis. Reprinted from the Primary Care Rheumatology Society.

date appraisal of current knowledge presented in the context of the implications for clinical management. The guidelines are intended to assist all health professionals in primary and secondary care who have a role in the management of patients treated with glucocorticoids.

References
1. Bone and Tooth Society, National Osteoporosis Society, Royal College of Physicians. Glucocorticoid-induced osteoporosis: guidelines for prevention and treatment. London: RCP, 2002.
2. Royal College of Physicians. Osteoporosis: clinical guidelines for prevention and treatment. London: RCP, 1999.

3. Royal College of Physicians, Bone and Tooth Society. Osteoporosis: clinical guidelines for prevention and treatment – Update on pharmacological interventions. London: RCP, 2000.

4. Department of Health. National service framework for older people. London: DH, 2001.

5. National Osteoporosis Society. Guidelines on the prevention and management of glucocorticoid osteoporosis. Bath: National Osteoporosis Society, 1998.

6. Department of Health. The new NHS: modern, dependable. London: Stationery Office, 1997.

7. Department of Health. Saving lives: our healthier nation. London: Stationery Office, 1999.

Summary guidance

- Glucocorticoids are widely used to treat a number of medical disorders. At any one time approximately 1% of the adult population in the UK is taking oral glucocorticoids; this figure increases to 2.4% in individuals aged 70–79 years (Level III).

- The administration of oral glucocorticoids is associated with a significant increase in fracture risk at the hip and spine (Level Ia). Although the greatest increase in risk is observed with higher dose therapy, increased risk is seen even at daily doses of prednisolone less than 7.5mg (Level III). Fracture risk increases rapidly after the onset of treatment and declines rapidly after stopping therapy (Level III).

- Loss of bone mineral density (BMD) associated with oral glucocorticoid administration is greatest in the first few months of glucocorticoid use (Level IIa). The effects of inhaled glucocorticoids on bone mineral density are less certain, although some studies report increased bone loss with high doses (Level IIa) and long-term use of lower doses may result in significant deficits of bone mineral density (Level III).

- Glucocorticoids contribute to the increase in fracture risk over and above the effect of low bone mineral density (Level Ia). Thus, for a given bone mineral density, the risk of fracture is higher in glucocorticoid-induced osteoporosis than in postmenopausal osteoporosis.

- Individuals at high risk, for example those aged 65 years or over and those with a prior fragility fracture, should be advised to commence bone-protective therapy at the time of starting glucocorticoids (Grade A). Measurement of bone density is not required before starting treatment.

- In other individuals, measurement of bone mineral density using dual energy X-ray absorptiometry is recommended for assessment of fracture risk in individuals treated with glucocorticoids (Grade C). Other secondary causes of osteoporosis should be excluded in individuals with a prior fracture (Grade C).
- General measures to reduce bone loss include reduction of the dose of glucocorticoids to a minimum, consideration of alternative formulations or routes of administration, and prescription of alternative immunosuppressive agents (Grade C). Good nutrition, an adequate dietary calcium intake and appropriate physical activity should be encouraged, and tobacco use and alcohol abuse avoided (Grade C).
- Evidence for the efficacy of agents in the prevention and treatment of glucocorticoid osteoporosis varies but beneficial effects on bone mineral density in the spine and hip have been demonstrated for several interventions (Level Ia). Fracture has not been a primary end-point of any studies of prevention or treatment of glucocorticoid-induced osteoporosis. Nevertheless, a reduction in vertebral fracture has been observed in post hoc or safety analyses of trials of etidronate, alendronate and risedronate (Level Ib).
- In other subjects receiving oral prednisolone, in whom it is intended to continue therapy for at least 3 months, bone densitometry should be considered (Grade C). A T score of –1.5 or lower may indicate the need for intervention with a bone-sparing agent (Level IV), although the effect of age on fracture probability in an individual should be taken into account when making treatment decisions (Grade C).
- The role of monitoring the effects of bone-protective agents in glucocorticoid-induced osteoporosis has not been established. However, significant treatment responses in some individuals may be detectable within one to two years by bone mineral density measurements in the spine (Level IV).

Extracted from: Bone and Tooth Society of Great Britain, National Osteoporosis Society, Royal College of Physicians. *Glucocorticoid-induced osteoporosis: guidelines for prevention and treatment.* London: RCP, 2002. Additional information is available at http://www.rcplondon.ac.uk and the full guidelines (*Glucocorticoid-induced osteoporosis: guidelines for prevention and treatment.* London: Royal College of Physicians, 2002) can be ordered from the Royal College of Physicians, 11 St Andrews Place, London NW1 4LE.

Clinical tools

WOMAC OA index

This 3-dimensional, self-administered measure specific to OA of the hip or knee uses either a visual analogue scale or a Likert scale to assess pain (5 questions), stiffness (2 questions) and physical function (17 questions). Details of the scale can be found in: Bellamy N, Buchanan WW, Goldsmith CH, et al. Validation study of WOMAC: a health status instrument for measuring clinically important patient relevant outcomes to antirheumatic drug therapy in patients with osteoarthritis of the hip or knee. *J Rheumatol* 1988;15:1833–40.

Chronic pain forms

The Glasgow NHS chronic pain forms are available from The Area Group for Chronic Pain, NHS Greater Glasgow (Tel: +44 (0)141 201 4000). The Royal Australian College of General Practitioners has Sharing Healthcare Guidelines for GPs in Chronic Condition Self Management Guideline. These are available from http://www.racgp.org.au/folder.asp?id=299.

Question, cue and response interview

Details of the question, cue and response interview can be found at http://som.flinders.edu.au/FUSA/CCTU/Home.html.

Numbers needed to treat

Adding codeine to paracetamol 600mg provides analgesia equivalent to a bigger (1g) dose of paracetamol, and paracetamol 1g with codeine 60mg is the best performer (Fig. 74). Extensive clinical experience attests that multiple dosing will show an even greater effect for patients with chronic pain. We know that the combinations work on different mechanisms to relieve pain. Although we could give the components separately, the convenience of just one medication is worthwhile, especially for elderly patients on many other drugs. Sustained-release morphine formulations are used (at huge cost) because they are perceived as more convenient. http://www.ebandolier.com

Use of analgesics

Details of the 3 pot system are available at http://www.ebandolier.com and in *Bandolier's Little Book of Pain* by Andrew Moore et al, Oxford University Press, ISBN 0-19-263247-7.

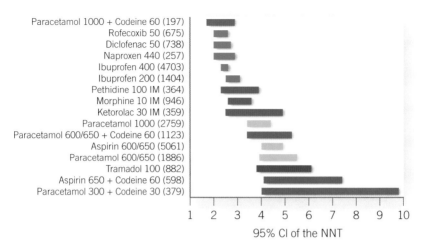

Fig. 74 League table
of number needed to
treat (NNT) for at least
50% pain relief over
4–6 hours in patients
with moderate to
severe pain.
Reprinted from
http://www.jr2.ox.ac.uk/
bandolier/booth/painpa
g/Acutrev/Analgesics/
Leagtab.html.

Stretching exercises for plantar fasciitis

The **arc** recommends these stretching exercises for patients with
Achilles tendonitis (1–3) and plantar fasciitis (1–4) (Fig. 75).

Exercise by Prescription

For questions about the *Exercise by Prescription* scheme, please phone
+44 (0)1642 444385.

Electronic booking

The electronic booking system for referrals to the Department of
Rheumatology at Guy's & St. Thomas' Hospital NHS Trust, London
was developed after consultation with GPs and rheumatologists at
King's College Hospital and at Guy's & St. Thomas'. The rheumatologist seeing the patient has an electronically printed letter of referral
with all the various details laid out in a formalized, standardized way
that makes for easy reading. Fig. 76 summarises the processes involved
in the electronic booking system.

1. Achilles tendon and plantar fascia stretch

First thing in the morning, loop a towel, a piece of elastic or a tubigrip around the ball of your foot and, keeping your knee straight, pull your toes towards your nose, holding for 30 seconds. Repeat 3 times for each foot.

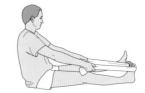

2. Wall push-ups or stretches for Achilles tendon

The Achilles tendon comes from the muscles at the back of your thigh and your calf muscles. These exercises need to be performed first with the knee **straight** and then with the knee **bent** in order to stretch both parts of the Achilles tendon. Twice a day do the following wall push-ups or stretches: (a) Face the wall, put both hands on the wall at shoulder height, and stagger the feet (one foot in front of the other). The front foot should be approximately 30 cm (12 inches) from the wall. With the front knee bent and the back knee straight, lean into the stretch (i.e., towards the wall) until a tightening is felt in the calf of the back leg, and then ease off. Repeat 10 times. (b) Now repeat this exercise but bring the back foot forward a little so that the back knee is slightly bent. Repeat the push-ups 10 times.

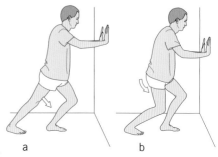

a   b

3. Stair stretches for Achilles tendon and plantar fascia

Holding the stair-rail for support, with legs slightly apart, position the feet so that both heels are off the end of the step. Lower the heels, keeping the knees straight, until a tightening is felt in the calf. Hold this position for 20–60 seconds and then raise the heels back to neutral. Repeat 6 times, at least twice a day.

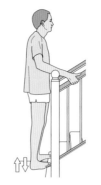

4. Dynamic stretches for plantar fascia

This involves rolling the arch of the foot over a rolling pin, a drinks can or a tennis ball, etc, while either standing (holding the back of a chair for support) or sitting. Allow the foot and ankle to move in all directions over the object. This can be done for a few minutes until there is some discomfort. Repeat this exercise at least twice a day. The discomfort can be relieved by rolling the foot on a cool drinks can from the fridge.

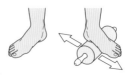

Fig. 75 Stretching exercises. Reproduced with kind permission from **arc** ("Hands On" Number 2 (HO2), February 2004). The exercise sheet can be downloaded from the **arc** website: www.arc.org.uk/about_arth/rdr5.htm.

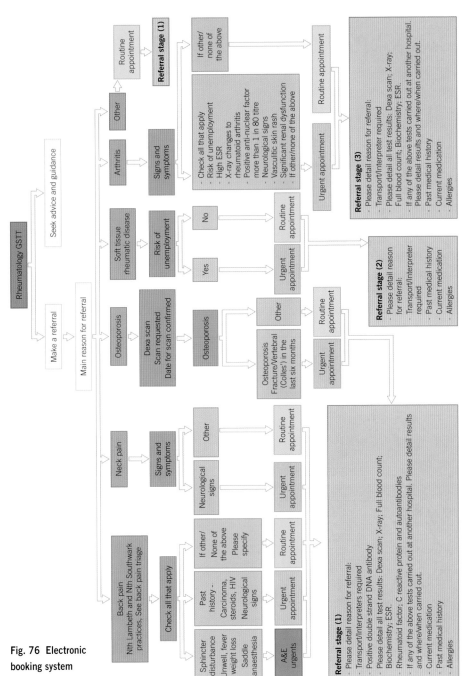

Fig. 76 Electronic booking system

Useful websites

http://som.flinders.edu.au/FUSA/CCTU/Home.html
The website of the Human Behaviour and Health Research Unit of
Flinders University, Australia, it deals with self-management of
chronic conditions.

www.arc.org.uk
Arthritis Research Campaign (**arc**) provides information for both
patients and physicians, as well as all the leaflets listed in appendix 7.

www.arthritiscare.org.uk
Arthritis Care offers self-help support, helpline service and a range of
leaflets on arthritis. Helplines: 020 7380 6555 (12–4pm, Mon–Fri) or
freephone: 0808 800 4050 (12–4pm, Mon–Fri).

www.mobilisphysiotherapy.com
Mobilis physiotherapy, provider of orthotics and physiotherapy products.

www.collegeofhealth.org.uk
The College of Health represents the interests of NHS patients.

www.dlf.org.uk
The Disabled Living Foundation (DLF) offers advice and information
on equipment to help with daily activities. Helpline: 0845 1330 9177
(10am–1pm, Mon–Fri).

www.doh.gov.uk/nsf/olderpeople/index.htm
The DOH website for Older People is intended primarily as a resource
for local NHS organizations and local councils to help in the implementation of the National Service Framework for Older People. It
may also be useful to older people and their carers.

www.ebandolier.com
Bandolier provides evidence-based thinking about healthcare. It
includes the Oxford Pain site.

www.jr2.ox.ac.uk/bandolier/painres/PRintro.html
Provides links to all resources available from Oxford Pain Research,
including material on arthritis.

www.eguidelines.co.uk/clip
This site contains all published guideline relevant to primary care.

www.eular.org
The European League Against Arthritis (EULAR) website provides up-to-date information in the field of rheumatology to allied health professionals, social leagues and patient organizations.

www.fleshandbones.com
Flesh and bones is a good resource for students.

www.healthsystem.virginia.edu/internet/familymed/docs/info_mastery.cfm
The Centre for Information Mastery from the Department of Family Medicine at the University of Virginia.

www.infopoems.com
POEMS, Patient-Orientated Evidence that Matters, address a question that we face as clinicians, measure outcomes that we and our patients care about: symptoms, morbidity, quality of life, and mortality, and have the potential to change the way we practice. This website, for InfoPOEMs (The Clinical Awareness System™), provides POEMs by subscription.

www.jointzone.org.uk
Jointzone is a comprehensive resource for physicians treating patients with joint problems.

www.move.uk.net
The MOVE (Making osteoarthritis matter) website provides older people with joint pain and locomotor disability with easily accessible and understandable information and information for health care professionals involved in the care of this client group.

www.nelh.nhs.uk/musculoskeletal
This MSK specialist library is a resource for all health care professionals working in the field of MSK medicine.

www.nice.org.uk
The National Institute for Clinical Excellence website contains previous appraisals and information on current appraisals of clinical treatments.

www.nlm.nih.gov/medlineplus/osteoporosis.html
Provided by the US National Library of Medicine and National Institutes of Health, this is a great resource for osteoporosis information.

www.nof.org/

The website of the US National Osteoporosis Foundation provides helpful information for both patients and physicians.

www.northglashealthinfo.org.uk

This is a comprehensive library resource for healthcare information.

www.osteo.org

This is the NIH osteoporosis website based in Washington, DC.

www.osteoporosis.ca

The **Osteoporosis Society of Canada** website has information to educate, empower and support individuals and communities in the prevention and treatment of osteoporosis.

www.painassociation.com

The Pain Association of Scotland provides support for people with chronic pain.

www.painconcern.org.uk

Pain Concern provides information and support for pain sufferers and those who care for them and about them.

www.painrelieffoundation.org.uk

The Pain Relief Foundation includes educational materials for healthcare professionals.

www.painsociety.org

The website of the Pain Society, the representative body for all professionals involved in the management and understanding of pain in the UK, provides pain scales in many languages.

www.pcrsociety.org.uk

The Primary Care Rheumatology Society (PCR) is a charity for doctors and other health professionals with an interest in musculoskeletal medicine. It provides education courses and is involved in research. Contact the executive secretary (Helen Livesley) at Helen@pcrsociety.freeserve.co.uk

www.racgp.org.au

The Royal Australian College of General Practice also deals with self-management of chronic conditions. It includes some very good booklets for doctors and health professionals that are well thought out and easy to follow.

www.rheumatoid.org.uk

The National Rheumatoid Arthritis Society (nras) has four main aims:
To provide an advisory and information service on all aspects of RA, to
raise public and government awareness of RA, to campaign for more
funding to be made available for treatment of the disease, and to facili-
tate the networking of patients and encourage self-help.

www.rheumatology.org

The American College of Rheumatology (ACR).

www.rheumatology.org.uk

The British Society of Rheumatology (BSR).

www.rsd-crps.co.uk

RSD UK is a patient support group for those with RSD or complex
regional pain syndrome.

www.thrive.org.uk *and* www.carryongardening.org.uk

Thrive provides information on easier gardening and a catalogue of
easy-to-use tools.

Especially for searching

www.bids.ac.uk

BIDS is a UK non-profit-making database provider that has access to
EMBASE.

www.bmn.com

The Biomednet databases include "evaluated" MEDLINE entries.

www.ncbi.nih.gov/PubMed

The Pub.Med database includes citations not yet on MEDLINE.

www.omni.ac.uk

OMNI, Organising Medical Networked Information, provides a search
engine for various websites and access to MEDLINE.

www.rccm.org.uk/ciscom

CISCOM is the Centralized Information Service for Complementary
Medicine.

Other patient support groups
Arthritis & Musculoskeletal Alliance (ARMA)
This alliance of professional and patient organizations can be found at 41 Eagle Street, London WC1R 4TL. Tel: +44 (0)20 7841 519.

Lupus UK
St. James House, Eastern Road, Romford, Essex RM1 3NH. Tel: +44 (0)1708 731251

The National Rheumatoid Arthritis Society (nras)
Briarwood House, 11 College Avenue, Maidenhead, Berkshire SL6 6AR, UK. Tel: 01628 670606; Fax: 01628 638810.

The British Sjögren's Syndrome Association
Unit 1 Manor Workshops, Nailsea Wall Lane, West End, Nailsea, Bristol BS19 2RA. Tel: +44 (0)1275 854215

The Raynaud's Scleroderma Association
112 Crewe Road, Alsager, Cheshire ST7 2JA. Tel: +44 (0)12708 72776

Useful publications
For patients
The Back Book. The Stationery Office, 2002, ISBN 0-11-322312-9.
Order from the Stationery Office, PO Box 29, Norwich NR3 1GN.
Tel: +44 (0)870 600 5522.

arc Patient information leaflets

Please see the **arc** website for a comprehensive list of leaflets and posters.

6018	A New Hip Joint	6103	Mind Map on Osteomalacia
6021	A New Knee Joint	6211	Mind Map Poster on Osteomalacia
6001	Ankylosing Spondylitis	6024	Neck pain
6059	Antiphospholipid Syndrome	6255	Occupational Therapy and Arthritis
6040	Are You Sitting Comfortably	6025	Osteoarthritis
6012	Arthritis and the Feet	6027	Osteoarthritis of the Knee
6054	Arthritis in Teenagers	6058	Osteomalacia
6002	Back Pain	6028	Osteoporosis
6003	Behcet's Syndrome	6031	Paget's Disease of the Bone
6004	Blood Tests and X-rays for Arthritis	6030	Pain and Arthritis
6005	Caring for a Person with Arthritis	6024	Pain in the Neck
6048	Carpal Tunnel Syndrome	6256	Physiotherapy and Arthritis
6038	Choosing Shoes	6032	Polymyalgia Rheumatica
6007	Complementary Therapies and Arthritis	6051	Pseudogout
6010	Diet and Arthritis	6029	Psoriatic Arthritis
6011	Driving and your Arthritis	6052	Raynaud's Syndrome
6250	Drugs for Arthritis: Local Steroid Injections	6034	Reactive Arthritis
6248	Drugs for Arthritis: NSAIDs	6035	Reflex Sympathetic Dystrophy
6253	Exercise and Arthritis	6036	Scleroderma
6013	Fibromyalgia	6037	Sexuality and Arthritis
6-014	Gardening with Arthritis	6056	Shoulder & Elbow Joint Replacements
6015	Gout	6041	Sjögren's Syndrome
6053	Growing Pains (written for children)	6042	Sports Injuries
6254	Hydrotherapy and Arthritis	6043	Stairlifts and Homelifts
6019	Hypermobility	6044	Tennis Elbow
6022	Knee Pain in Young Adults	6039	The Painful Shoulder
6055	Looking after your Joints when you have RA	6047	Vasculitis
6023	Lupus (SLE)	6262	Work and Arthritis
6101	Mind Map on Gout	6049	Work Related Rheumatic Complaints
		6017	Your Home and your Rheumatism

For health professionals
arc In Practice and Topical Reviews for Health Professionals

No.10	A General Practice Approach to Management of Chronic Widespread Musculoskeletal Pain and Fibromyalgia.
6509	Chronic Pain: A Primary Care Condition
6503	Connective Tissue Diseases and the Role of the GP
6505	Corticosteroid Induced Osteoporosis
6501	Cox-2 for General Practitioners
6506	Modern Podiatry
6507	Neck Pain (Cervical Spondylosis)
6504	OA of the Knee and Hip
6609	OA Risk Factors and Pathogenesis
6601	Osteoporosis and Metabolic Bone Disease
6602	Polymyalgia Rheumatica
6511	Preventing and Managing Chronic Disability
6606	Rheumatic Diseases Associated with Antinuclear Antibodies
6604	Seronegative Spondarthritis
6502	Shoulder Problems
6607	Use of Analgesics in Rheumatology
6510	Widespread Musculoskeletal Pain and Fibromyalgia

arc Hands on for Health Professionals

No. 1	PMR
No. 2	Plantar fasciitis
No. 3	Carpal tunnel syndrome

Further reading

Hochberg MC, Silman, Smolen, Weinblatt & Weisman.
Rheumatology, 3rd ed. Edinburgh: Mosby, 2003.

Dieppe P, Paine T. Referral guidelines for general practitioners: which
patients with limb joint arthritis should be sent to a rheumatologist? *arc Reports Series* 1994;3:6331.

Ahmad Y, Bruce I. Connective tissue diseases and the role of the general practitioner. *arc Reports Series* 2003;4:6503.

Watts RA, Scott DGI. Primary systemic vasculitis. *Rheumatic Disease
Topical Reviews* 2003:no. 11.

Symmons D, Asten P, McMally R. *Healthcare Needs Assessment for
Musculoskeletal Diseases. The First Step – Estimating the Number of
Incident and Prevalent Cases*, 2nd ed. Arthritis Research Campaign,
2002.

Arthritis – The Big Picture. Arthritis Research Campaign, 2002.
Obtainable from **arc**.

Evidence-based management initiatives

Faculty of Health Sciences, University of Queensland, Australia
(www.uq.edu.au) has prepared a document that focuses on treatment of pain in five areas: lower back, neck, thoracic spine, knee
and shoulder. The document can be viewed and comments made
online at www.uq.edu.au/health/msp.

Shoulder pain

Hay EM, Thomas E, Paterson SM, et al. A pragmatic randomised
controlled trial of local corticosteroid injection and physiotherapy
for the treatment of new episodes of unilateral shoulder pain in
primary care. *Ann Rheum Dis* 2003;**62**:394–9.

Winters JC, Sobel JS, Groenier KH, et al. Comparison of physiotherapy, manipulation, and corticosteroid injection for treating shoulder complaints in general practice: randomised, single blind study.
BMJ 1997;**314**:1320–5.

van der Windt DA, Koes BW, Deville W, et al. Effectiveness of corticosteroid injections versus physiotherapy for treatment of painful
stiff shoulder in primary care: randomised trial. *BMJ*
1998;**317**:1292–6.

Carpal tunnel syndrome

Katz JN, Simmons BP. Clinical practice. Carpal tunnel syndrome.
NEJM 2002;**346**:1807–12.

Tennis/golfers elbow

Smidt N, van der Windt DAWM, Assendelft WJJ, et al. Corticosteroid injections, physiotherapy, or a wait-and-see policy for lateral epicondylitis: a randomised controlled trial. *Lancet* 2002;**359**:657–62.

Patella taping

Cushnaghan J, McCarthy C, Dieppe P. Taping the patella medially: a new treatment for OA of the knee joint? *BMJ* 1994;**308**:753–5.

Hinman RS, Bennell KL, Crossley KM, et al. Immediate effects of adhesive tape on pain and disability in individuals with knee osteoarthritis. *Rheumatology* 2003;**42**:865–9.

Topical NSAIDs

Moore RA, Tramer MR, Carroll D, et al. Quantitative systematic review of topically applied non-steroidal anti-inflammatory drugs. *BMJ* 1998;**316**:333–8.

Joint replacement

Fortin PR, Clarke AE, Joseph L, et al. Outcomes of total hip and knee replacement: preoperative functional status predicts outcomes at six months after surgery. *Arthritis Rheum* 1999;**42**:1722–8.

Nilsdotter AK, Petersson IF, Roos EM, et al. Predictors of patient relevant outcome after total hip replacement for osteoarthritis: a prospective study. *Ann Rheum Dis* 2003;**62**:923–30.

Negret P, Donnell ST, Dejour H. Osteoarthritis of the knee following meniscectomy. *BJR* 1994;**33**;367–8.

Roos H, Lauren M, Roos EM, et al. Risk factors and osteoarthrosis after meniscectomy. *Arthitis Rheum* 1998;**41**(**suppl 9**):abstract 326.

Osteomalacia

Nellen JFJB, Smulders YM, Jos Frissen PH, et al. Hypovitaminosis D in immigrant women: slow to be diagnosed. *BMJ* 1996;**312**:570–2.

Index

Note: As the subject of this book is arthritis, all entries refer to arthritis unless stated. Page numbers in *italics* refer to figures and/or tables.

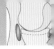

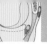

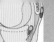